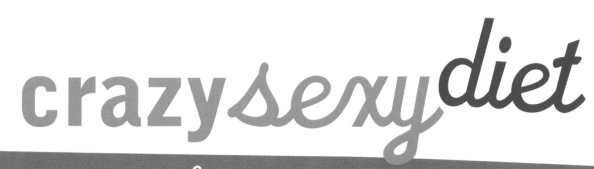

crazy sexy diet

Eat your veggies, ignite your spark, and live like you mean it!

kris carr

skirt!

Guilford, Connecticut
An imprint of Globe Pequot Press

skirt! is an attitude . . . spirited, independent,
outspoken, serious, playful and irreverent,
sometimes controversial, always passionate.

Text design and layout: Karla Baker
Project editor: Kristen Mellitt
Nutrition consultant: Jennifer K. Reilly, RD
Culinary expert and chef contributor: Chad Sarno

Library of Congress Cataloging-in-Publication Data is
available on file.

ISBN 978-1-59921-801-4

Printed in the United States of America

10 9 8 7 6 5 4 3 2 1

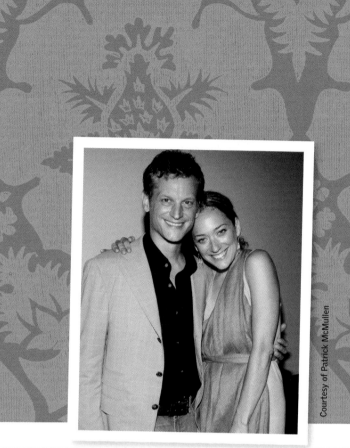

Courtesy of Patrick McMullen

For my talented husband, Brian, you are my North

Star, my muse, and my mentor. Without your support

(and brilliant edits) this book would still be in my head.

Thank you for your endless guidance and for helping

me become the woman I always wanted to be. I will

love you unconditionally for many lifetimes.

Contents

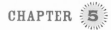
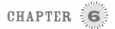
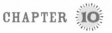

BE AN ACTIVE PARTICIPANT
IN YOUR HEALTH
Dr. Dean Ornish

I love Kris Carr. She *glows*.

It's not just because of what she's done, which is extraordinary. It's who she is.

Faced with an overwhelming cancer diagnosis, Kris grabbed the reins and became a voracious student of all things health and wellness. She transformed her life and became a shining example of an "empowered participant" in her body, mind, and spiritual health. She was able to integrate the best of modern medicine and ancient healing traditions to transform a diagnosis of death into vibrant living.

Many patients have told me, "Being diagnosed with cancer was the best thing that ever happened to me." A skeptic might reply, "What are you, crazy?" To which they might hear, "That's what it took to get my attention to begin changing my life in ways that have made it so much more joyful and meaningful."

Not that we look for illness or suffering, but sometimes, for reasons that may be a mystery, there it is. What we do with it makes all the difference in the world. Even when we can't be cured, we can be healed, becoming more whole. When we become active participants in our healing, it may bring meaning to our suffering, which makes it more bearable. Often, our physical illnesses improve as well.

Change is hard. But if we're in enough pain, the idea of change becomes more appealing—"Well, it may be hard to change my diet and lifestyle, but I'm in so much pain I'm willing to try something different."

In 2009, the Nobel Prize in Medicine went to Dr. Elizabeth Blackburn for discovering telomerase, an enzyme that repairs and lengthens damaged telomeres, which are the ends of our chromosomes that control aging. Dr. Blackburn and her colleague, Dr. Elissa Epel, studied women who were under chronic emotional stress because they were taking care of children with autism or chronic diseases.

They found that the more stressed the women felt, and the longer they felt stressed, the lower was their telomerase and the shorter their telomeres. This was the first study providing genetic evidence indicating that chronic emotional stress might shorten a woman's lifespan.

What was particularly interesting to me was that it wasn't an objective measure of stress that determined the effects on their telomeres; it was the women's perception of stress that mattered. In other words, two women might be in comparable situations, but one had learned to manage her stress better by empowering herself and taking charge of her life. As a result, her telomeres were longer.

We tend to think of advances in medicine as a new drug, laser, surgical procedure—something high-tech and expensive. We often have a hard time believing that the simple choices that we make in our lives each day—what we eat, how we respond to stress, how much exercise we get, and (perhaps most important), how much love and intimacy we have—can make such a powerful difference in our health and well-being, but they do.

For more than thirty-three years, my colleagues and I at the non-profit Preventive Medicine Research Institute and the School of Medicine, University of California–San Francisco have conducted a series of studies showing that what was once thought impossible was often achievable.

We found that a whole foods, plant-based diet (such as the one described in this book), moderate exercise, stress management techniques such as yoga and meditation, and learning to give and receive love more fully (what we euphemistically call "social support") could often reverse the progression of coronary heart disease, early-stage prostate cancer, type 2 diabetes, high blood pressure, hypercholesterolemia, obesity, depression, and other chronic diseases.

We found that changing your lifestyle changes your genes. So often, I hear people say, "Oh, it's all in my genes, there's not much I can do about it," what I call "genetic nihilism." In men with prostate cancer, we found that making these comprehensive lifestyle changes for only three months caused changes in over five hundred genes—"turning on" disease-preventing genes and "turning off" genes that promote many chronic diseases, including a series of oncogenes that promote breast cancer, colon cancer, and prostate cancer.

Your genes are a predisposition, but your genes are not your fate.

Along with Dr. Blackburn, we also measured telomerase levels in these patients. We found that telomerase increased by almost 30 percent in only three months. And while comprehensive lifestyle changes may increase telomerase, even drugs have not yet been shown to do this.

These studies are empowering many people with new hope and new choices.

So is Kris Carr.

Joy, pleasure, and freedom are sustainable. Because the mechanisms that affect our health are so much more dynamic than had once been realized, most people find that when they make the lifestyle changes described in this book, they feel so much better, so quickly, it reframes the reason for change from fear of dying (which is not sustainable) to joy of living (which is).

These are the practices Kris lays out so intelligently and simply in *Crazy Sexy Diet*. And not only this—she also explains in clear, layman's language the science and logic behind these choices. Why should we eat plant-based foods? Why are whole grains superior to processed ones, and which ones are superior to others? How much protein, fat, and sugar do we really need, and how do we go about getting them without the excessive consumption of animal products?

Consider this not a diet book, but a guide to living fully; not a meal plan, but a road map to self-empowerment, adorned with Kris's unrivaled enthusiasm, humor, and compassion.

And by the time you finish this book, there's a good chance you may love Kris, too.

Dean Ornish, MD is the founder and president of the Preventive Medicine Research Institute (www.pmri.org) and Clinical Professor of Medicine at the University of California–San Francisco.

YOUR WHOLE LIFE
IS ABOUT TO BE AMAZING!
Rory Freedman

If you look around, you may notice

that many among us in the human race are sleepwalking through life. Friends, family members, the masses—it's incredibly common and incredibly sad. And if you look at yourself, you may notice that you too are among the living dead. You may be tempted to ask, "How did this happen? How long has it been going on for? How did I get here?"

Who cares? Life is short! Don't waste another second in no-man's land! That Kris's book landed in your lap is no coincidence—it is actually a miracle. It's a miracle because it's the key to the rest of your life, which starts NOW!

There are few things you can do to impact your life more powerfully, profoundly, and permanently than changing your diet. Every morsel of food that enters your mouth has a direct impact on your body, mind, and spirit. I learned this firsthand when I changed my own diet in 1994. Not only did my body change, but I felt happier, healthier, and more positive then ever before. Something shifted inside me that I never expected or even thought to look for. But there it was. Changing my diet changed my world and completely changed who I was. And it only improved from there. (My best-selling book, *Skinny Bitch,* was born from that change, btw.) Today, I credit everything good in my life to this dietary shift and

cannot imagine who I would be had I not seen the light that fateful day. And now, today is your day. That you have all this empowering, compelling information directly from Crazy, Sexy Kris Carr, Unicorn Goddess, is truly a blessing. Do not squander it, mortal! You too can be a unicorn. All you need to do is take the first step. Get excited. Pee a little. This is huge! YOUR WHOLE LIFE IS ABOUT TO BE AMAZING.

First order of business: Create a reasonable, yet challenging, goal for yourself with regards to your new eating plan. It can be as basic as "no soda" or as advanced as "totally vegan." You decide what you're up for and what you can handle. But definitely stretch yourself a little beyond your comfort zone. When you figure out what you're gonna do, then figure out the when. Set a date in the next few weeks, and commit to trying twenty-one days with this new lifestyle. Be smart about when you start—birthdays and holidays aren't the easiest times to change your ways. And be conscientious of the language you use when staking your new dietary claims. Keep it positive and productive. For example: "I'm going to treat my temple to water instead of toxic soda for the next twenty-one days," as opposed to, "I have to give up soda for a month . . . how am I gonna live?"

Phase two: Enlist a friend. There is nothing better than having support and camaraderie when tackling a goal. In mid-October 2009, I decided to go until Thanksgiving without eating any sugar. Six weeks with no dessert. FRESH HELL. (I'm allowed to use negative language since I already conquered my goal. I make the rules.) The first thing I did was recruit two friends to do it with me. And within a few days of starting the cleanse, I recruited three more. While we griped, groaned, and suffered, we did it all together. Three weeks in, one friend hit an emotional bottom and tried to bail out. But we were all there to lean on and he finished successfully with the rest of us. When it was all said and done, two from our sugar-free group felt so amazing, they stuck with it even after the cleanse was over. So choose at least one friend (but hopefully a few) who you know will be up for the challenge, will support you when you're down, and who won't let you quit on yourself.

Mach three: Get prepared. Clear all the crap out of your kitchen, stock your fridge and pantry with the right foods, and map out an eating plan to get you through the month. (Kris shows you how.) Have fun with it. Check out new cookbooks, go online for recipes, plan potlucks with friends. You can eat well and enjoy food. And you should!

Final phase: The pinky promise. With enrolled friend, look in each other's eyes and shake pinkies to seal the deal. State out loud what your intentions are and your start and stop dates—to yourselves, to each other, to the Universe. This is real. This is a binding contract between you and your friend, you and the Universe, and most important, you and yourself. This is the beautiful, exciting, and exhilarating place where the rubber meets the road. This is where magic truly and really happens. This is where you actually CHANGE your LIFE!

Rory Freedman is a vegan and animal rights activist and coauthor of the best-seller *Skinny Bitch*.

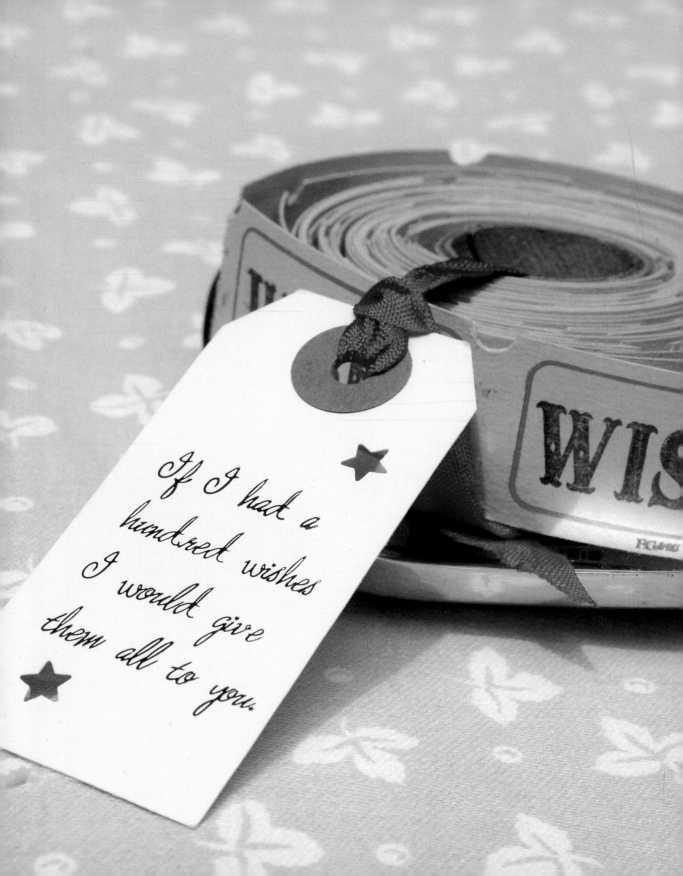

THIS IS YOUR
WAKE-UP CALL
pick up, gorgeous!

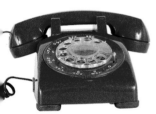

Are you ready to live like you mean it? Are you ready to get out of your slump, over your fear, and plug into your Crazy Sexy potential? For those of you who are new to the Crazy Sexy concept, let me lay it out for you. Crazy = bold, out of the box, forward thinking, and status quo challenging. Sexy = confident, in touch, whole, passionate, and conscious. Sound good? Well, the Crazy Sexy red phone is ringing—loud and clear. Pick up, gorgeous!

At some point in our lives, every one of us dazzling human beings clomping around in heels gets an important call from the "This Is Your Chance" hotline. For some, like me, the entry point came in the form of medical desperation. Life hits a 911 tipping point and suddenly you're up against the ropes of mortality, begging for one more shot. You realize that the only way to get out of the rubble is to rebuild a more sustainable you.

For others, a divine disco light ignites the spark and your third eye explodes with love for yourself. In that instant your inner Queen wakes up to the holy "Wow, I'm worth it" truth. Good-bye, woe-is-me thinking, and hello, royal care. The awakening is like a cosmic consciousness cocktail that makes you tipsy with self-empowerment.

Or maybe it's not quite so dramatic and extreme. Maybe your call to action comes from boredom or just feeling "over it." You're literally

Say What? crazy sexy DIET?

Let me lay it out for you: The Crazy Sexy Diet is a low-fat, vegetarian—or better yet, vegan—program that emphasizes balancing your body's pH by eating more lush whole foods, low-glycemic fruits, raw veggies, alkalizing green drinks, and super-powered green smoothies. By increasing the amount of alkaline foods you eat while decreasing acidic foods (animal products, processed sugars and starches, etc.), you reduce inflammation and boost immunity and life force. In short, you stack the good-health odds in your favor. Hip hip hooray!

The Crazy Sexy Diet has two flexible levels, which you can slide between depending on your needs and lifestyle: 60/40 and 80/20: 60 or 80 percent alkaline foods, 40 or 20 percent acidic. While 80/20 is optimum, 60/40 is a healthy balance for long-term maintenance. If you're already in good health, you will see amazing results with this ratio. The 80/20 ratio is advised for those of you who have been or are living with a disease or illness, or who simply want to go for the gold-standard diet. But let's get one thing straight up front: These ratios do not refer to 60 percent healthy food, 40 percent junk from the candy, chip, and Slim Jim aisle. It's all whole food. Lots of it is raw, some of it is cooked, but none of it's crappy. And as you'll learn, my definition of crappy may be very different from yours.

To kick off the CSD, after learning all there is to know about it, you'll have the opportunity to set sail on a 21-Day Cleanse filled with juicy goodness, plenty of produce, and no stinky dead stuff. Not only that, but I've packed it with inspiration, affirmations, strong intentions, prayer beads, and some practical tips to kick your beautiful butt and get you into glorious high gear!

sick and tired of being sick and tired. No more marking time. No more sofas, remotes, and stalking people on Facebook. No more excuses. Amen, sister!

Regardless of how you arrived here, you're farther along than you think. Just by picking up this book, you've proved that you have what it takes to become a kick-ass Wellness Warrior. Let's give you the body and soul makeover you deserve! It's time to clear the slate and get back to basics. Like the Bionic Woman, you will be stronger, faster, and have great hair, but only if you smarten up and change your life. Stop mainlining stress or pile-driving Cinnabons and get with the Crazy Sexy program, lady!

Do you have any idea what it's like to feel blissfully whole and comfortable in your skin? Do you know what it's like to be centered and grounded yet filled with an abundant supply of zippy energy? You will. The Crazy Sexy Diet and lifestyle (otherwise known as CSD) gives you the tools to navigate your journey with clarity and balance. There are many things that are out of your control (your neighbor's bratty kid,

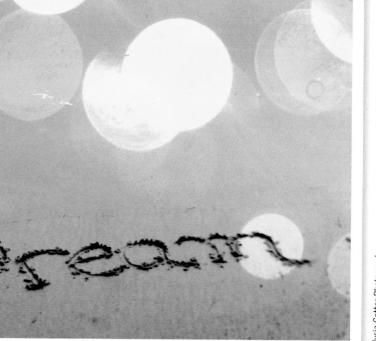

rainstorms, skinny jeans and tube tops), yet you actually have a lot of power over your health, happiness, and life—and it all starts with your mouth. What you put in it, and the words that come out of it, determine your destiny. Shitty nutrition and chemical crutches will wear you out. Stinkin' thinkin' and verbal self-abuse amputate your angel wings.

Health is more than just the absence of disease; it is the presence of vitality. Health is freedom from obstruction; it's living in a harmonious way that creates both inner and outer peace. Change the menu. Rewrite the recipe and break your bad eating habits before they break you. The perception that optimum well-being is beyond our reach enables us to avoid taking responsibility for our lifestyle choices. But when you focus on what you consume literally (food and drink) and figuratively (thoughts, ideas, gossip, bad reality TV)—your world transforms at the deepest level. Saying yes to yourself creates an auspicious shift in other areas of your life. A new job,

passion, or cause presents itself. An abandoned dream gets a second shot. Fulfilling relationships replace one-way streets. A health issue stabilizes and in some cases reverses. One thing is certain: Gorgeous you will glimmer inside and out.

Nobody can take away your ruby shine when you're happy and healthy. And when you're in that positive space, there's a cascade effect: You pay it forward by sharing your wellness tips through deed and example. It's a win–win situation. But there's more. Your choices are not only terrific for you, they're awesome for the planet. Holy hip shake, that's cool!

CRAZY = bold, out of the box, forward thinking, and status quo challenging.

SEXY = confident, in touch, whole, passionate, and conscious.

OH MY GOD!
I can't believe I'm writing a DIET BOOK!

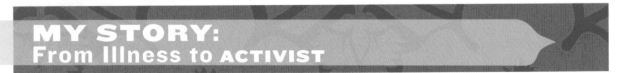

To be honest, my dream was never to create another diet book. Especially because "diets" don't always work! Yet I couldn't keep my years of research and experimentation to myself. As a result of the success of my documentary film *Crazy Sexy Cancer* (which I wrote and directed for TLC) and my first two books, *Crazy Sexy Cancer Tips* and *Crazy Sexy Cancer Survivor,* so many people wrote to ask me what I eat, how to meditate, what books to read, where to go for detoxification or wellness retreats, and how to best balance it all. These letters didn't just come from cancer patients—curious seekers from around the world who were looking to make healthy changes in their lives also reached out to me. These motivated mystics gravitated to my anything-is-possible attitude and real-deal information.

The program I lay out for you in this book encompasses far more than diet, it's the overall lifestyle that works for me and countless other people. While I am not a doctor or a scientist, I am a Crazy Sexy survivor. Since changing what I eat and how I live, my body and mind are healthy, strong, and empowered. I prove my own point every day, and the proof is definitely in the pudding. This is why I have included some inspirational testimonials from folks who have adopted my lifestyle. Their stories are as powerful as the people who share them. Join us!

In these challenging times it's crucial to become "Prevention Is Hot" cheerleaders. Set an example, teach your children, and lead the way to health, spiritual wealth, and happiness through personal action. Nobody knows your body like you do, and waiting around for someone else to fix your woes is playing a risky game of roulette.

This book is my gift to you, a love letter to life born from a crappy diagnosis that became the catalyst for a healthier existence. You'll read some of the details of my mud in a minute. But hey, no mud, no lotus, right? The most beautiful things spring from the compost pile. Cancer rocked my world and forced me to find a "new normal." The Crazy Sexy Diet is the result of my years of questioning and study—it's loaded with information that will deeply transform your life and possibly even save it—or at the very least reduce the pesky cellulite! It's an awakening without the disease, knowledge without the price. Changing your mind may be the biggest obstacle you face. But once you do, you'll realize that you are the one you've been waiting for . . .

MY STORY:
From Illness to ACTIVIST

My wake-up call came on February 14, 2003. "Happy Valentine's Day, you have canSer"—spelled wrong to piss it off and take my power back. At the time I was a fabulous thirty-one-year-old actress and photographer living in New York City. Actually, I was a party hound and stress slut, trying to get my shit together and make a name for myself. Sometimes I lived high on the hog; other times I could barely put the fast food on the table. That's kinda the nature of the arts: feast or famine. On my personal D-Day, I found myself lying on a cold exam table while a nurse named Mildred passed an ultrasound scanner across my belly. Piercing abdominal cramps and shortness of breath had forced me back to my primary care doctor. It was the same pain I had felt for three years, only magnified. Since my doctor hadn't found anything wrong with me on the previous visits, I learned to live with the discomfort. "You're like most uptight city girls," he said. "Constipated!" Plus, I had Teflon youth on my side: Nothing could happen to me. Yet on that particular day the pain was unbearable. I figured I'd blown it out a few weeks before while partying at a film festival where a movie I was in premiered. Showing off for a hot dude in yoga class probably didn't help, either.

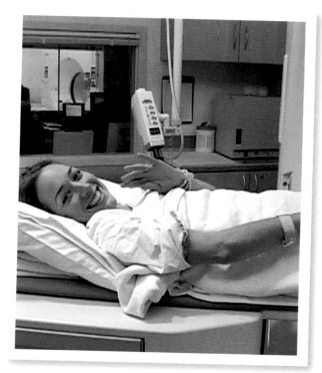

    The nurse's distressed look forced me to ask her what she saw. "I can't tell you that," she sternly replied. "You'll have to speak with the doctor." Okay, I could wait a few more minutes. In walks the doctor. "The surface of your liver is covered with about a dozen lesions," he said. I had no idea what that meant. I thought lesions meant cuts and I wondered how I'd cut my liver. Yes, I regularly enjoyed a few cocktails and other recreational substances, but wasn't this an extreme result of a few indiscretions?

    Then he clarified things for me. The lesions were tumors, a twelve-pack of misery that made the ultrasound images of my liver look like Swiss cheese. But that wasn't all; about ten more tumors were in my lungs. And get this, the cancer was completely inoperable, no surgery, radiation, chemotherapy, and—here's the knockout punch—no cure! In an instant I went from hot chick to sick chick, saddled with an extremely rare sarcoma called epithelioid hemangioendothelioma (EHE) that affects less than 0.01 percent of the cancer population. Little is known about

my annoyingly hard-to-spell and -pronounce disease, and none of the big C cancer bucks go into studying it. Whiskey Tango Foxtrot (that's military speak for "what the fuck?").

BAD LIVER

This must be a joke, I thought. I had no medical history of cancer. I was barely a day over thirty-one and single, which to me meant that my freelance dating career was now officially over. No more opportunities to taste a bunch of appetizers without having to commit to one main course. It was sexual fasting time. My life was stigmatized and shattered. Friends dumped me, colleagues stepped back as if I had some contagious plague, and the "So sorry to hear you're dying" sympathy cards started pouring in.

    How did this happen? I was good, I followed the rules, I didn't jaywalk or rob banks, I exercised, drank in moderation-ish, ate "right" from time to time, I said please, thank you, tipped 20 percent. For God's sake, I was a Democrat and a Bud girl!

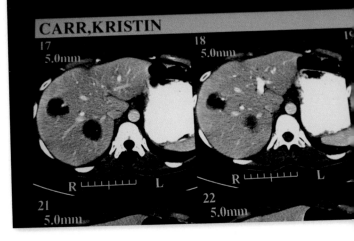

Second and third opinions, along with endless hours at the University of Google, followed. I quickly learned that illness was a business, and if I wanted to successfully navigate hurricane cancer, I needed to take my emotions out of it. Good-bye Broadway. Hello CEO of Save My Ass Technologies, Inc.! I was the CEO, and the doctors worked for me. In order to survive I needed to staff up posthaste.

The job description read something like this:

FREAKED-OUT PATIENT SEEKS BRILLIANT ONCOLOGIST WHO KNOWS ABSOLUTELY EVERYTHING THERE IS TO KNOW ABOUT HER EXTREMELY RARE AND RIDICULOUS DISEASE.

```
Must be a geeky scientist with
his or her finger on the pulse
of the latest cutting-edge treat-
ments. Team players only. No
my-way-or-the-highway-one-size-
fits-all-nonsense will be toler-
ated. A pleasant bedside manner
is mandatory. No Hell's Angels
or military strategists, please.
Those applicants with degrees
from trade schools located some-
where in the Caribbean need not
apply.
```

There were a few qualified applicants, as well as a bunch of duds. The doctor who suggested a triple organ transplant was rejected immediately. I mean, how rude! The one who gave me ten years to live can still kiss my ass. Though I knew I was in a shit storm, I still didn't know how quickly the cancer was moving. So pulling out organs, blasting my body with chemicals, or dying seemed a bit premature. It was clear that I would have to advocate for myself and learn how to navigate the system.

I traveled everywhere searching for my second in command and finally found him. Honestly, if it weren't for my oncologist, I might not be here today. Guess what he confirmed? The cancer was slow moving, so in essence I had the one thing all cancer patients long for—time. This was great news, and because of it I chose a radical course of treatment: Do nothing. He agreed.

"We'll take a watch-and-wait approach," he said. "Let cancer make the first move."

Great! But how about a watch-and-live approach? And what if I made the first move?

If I couldn't be cured, could I still be healthy? Could wellness be redefined to include someone like me? Perhaps instead of calling it cancer, I would call it imbalance. And what if I could find the source of the imbalance? Maybe, just maybe, I could help my body and my mind keep the disease in check. Clearly, I had a lot to learn, but joy came back, and curiosity started bubbling. This wouldn't be my battle: It would be the greatest adventure of my life.

Could wellness be redefined to include someone like me?

ENTER THE INNER MD

Through some down-and-dirty personal exploration, I met my Inner Physician. She's smart, curious, and highly intuitive (plus she looks lovely in a white coat). The prescription she offered was quite simple. "Renovate your life, kiddo. Be a self-reliant detective and put the pieces of your health puzzle together." Suddenly I felt like one of Charlie's Angels. Would any of them crumble under pressure? No! They'd put on a cute outfit, some gloss, and get down to business. My Inner MD encouraged me to collaborate with my body, to work on simpler things that would make a profound difference. In order to do that, I had to get the hell out of the way so my body could regain homeostasis.

Because my diet had been based on what to eat to stay slim for the camera, I had no idea how to be healthy. I'd spend endless energy weighing my food and counting calories and fat grams. Meals were planned around convenience, auditions, and cocktail hour. My mantra: Unwrap, nuke, GO! Vegetables were far too elegant and way too time consuming to buy and make at home. Fake foods encased in plastic or cardboard were time-effective and cheap. The multisyllabic poisons on the label didn't scare me. I figured, "If it was dangerous they would never sell it to me. Doesn't the FDA ban the bad stuff?" Besides, all I cared about was the promise on the package. "Look great and lose weight while still enjoying this sensible cake." I could eat this crap and my ass would be teeny-weeny. Hallelujah!

The early signs and symptoms were obvious, but I couldn't see them for what they were: a toxic lifestyle and environment that was causing physical and emotional stress. I had a bunch of chronic health problems, including zits, colds, chest infections, allergies, depression (Prozac and wine helped that), dry skin, eczema, low sex drive (in my twenties!), bloating, constipation, abdominal pain, acid reflux, yeast infections, and fatigue—all distress signals from an imbalanced body. Yet rather than dealing with the real issues in my tissues, I'd often compound the problem by tossing drugs down my

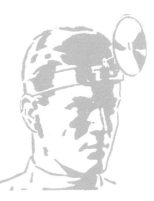

gullet. Over time, my symptoms worsened until they became unbearable. Obviously, I needed to make some changes.

Next stop: Whole Foods, my new pharmacy. In the beginning, I had no idea what I was doing. I would race around the store frantically filling shopping carts with books, videos, supplements, powders, potions, and every piece of organic produce I could get my hands on. Kale? Okay! It was dark green and leafy, so it must be good for me. Yet in the back of my mind I wondered what the heck I'd do with this scary-looking weed. If the cancer didn't kill me, this plant certainly might.

I made a checklist of my physical problems and began working on them. I addressed my insomnia and taught myself how to sleep. Practices like meditation helped me deal with the wild animals in my head. I learned that my excuses for not exercising were really lame. If you're like me, you max out your time and leave nothing left for sweat. Earth to us: A regular exercise plan is not optional. It heals our bodies, calms our minds, and gives us the energy we need to kick ass.

I went back to school to study nutrition so that I could finally learn how to eat and take care of myself! Fuck geometry, I'll take nutrition any day. I also quit my acting career, sold my apartment, and became a full-time healing junkie (with certifications). After trading in my fast-paced New York City party life for snail-pace living at a Zen monastery in New Mexico, I finally settled on a simple, nature-filled existence in Woodstock, New York. I exchanged road rage for prayer, fast food for fasting, swapped martinis for organic green drinks and a compassionate vegan diet.

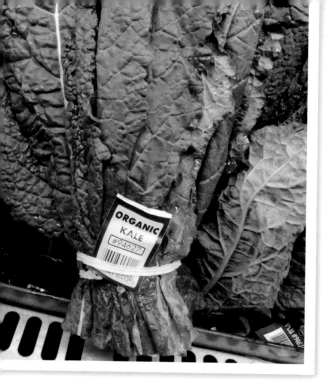

really matter. The fact is, my blood work is fantastic, I have endless energy, my immune system is strong, and (drumroll) . . . I'm happy! That's right, happy.

In this Crazy Sexy book you'll learn the secrets that have helped me thrive in the face of a deadly chronic disease. Imagine what they can do for you. Sorry, I don't mean to brag, but there is one more thing and if you're a love-hunting (bad-relationship-finding) lady like I was, it might inspire you to know that I found my soul mate after my diagnosis demanded I change. So much for "damaged goods." I married the editor of my film. Cancer or not, when I dumped the junk and aligned myself with my higher purpose, the pieces of the puzzle fell into place. There's no need to wait for the bad things and bullshit to be over. Change now. Love now. Live now. Don't wait for people to give you permission to live, because they won't. That permission is your birthright, hot stuff; grab it!

Seven years later I still have cancer, but it's stable. My beauty marks, as I call them, lie dormant. But thanks to my diet and lifestyle I feel and look better than I ever have in my life (even before my diagnosis). Whether my success is due to the nature of my disease or the nature of my choices doesn't

Change now.
Love now.
Live now.

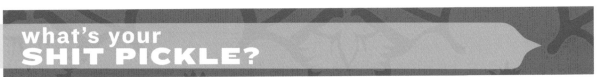

what's your
SHIT PICKLE?

So . . . what's your cancer? Are you overweight, depressed? Do you have heart disease or diabetes? Is your cholesterol too high? How about regret, procrastination, or maybe even a crazy (not-so-sexy) divorce? What the shit pickle happens to be doesn't really matter; it's what you do with it that will transform your life. Let it be your guru rather than your jailer. Let it ignite your gut wisdom and introduce yourself to your own Inner MD. She'll straighten you up just like mine did.

Here's where diet and lifestyle choices really matter. To hear that voice, you must strip away the garbage. You can't get clear when you're running on Lucky Charms consciousness. Meet your genetic potential by shifting what you eat and how you think about food—that's where the Crazy Sexy Diet comes in. Think of the diet as your Inner MD's medical assistant.

Don't get down on yourself. Remember we've all got our own version of cancer—even the seemingly

Perfect 10 girl who lives in the next condo. Lucky you that you realize it and are willing to do something. More than half of all Americans die of heart disease or cancer; two-thirds are overweight and stay that way for their whole lives. We are one of the wealthiest countries in the world and yet we're ranked number thirty-three in health care (behind Slovenia). When I was in grade school, my friends weren't getting adult diseases like Type 2 diabetes, nor were we doped up on behavioral medications. Everyone ate their peas and drank an extra glass of OJ when they had the sniffles. If someone had restless leg syndrome, they were told to take a walk!

In the United States we spend more on sickness than wellness. Young people are being diagnosed with catastrophic diseases common among their grandparents. Some medical researchers say that the next generation will be the first generation to die younger than their parents. The solution is clear as far as I'm concerned: Combine the latest reliable science with smart nutrition and positive lifestyle changes. So as our brilliant doctors continue to break new ground, we must meet them halfway by improving our diet and lifestyle choices, controlling stress, and cleaning up our environment in order to stay well.

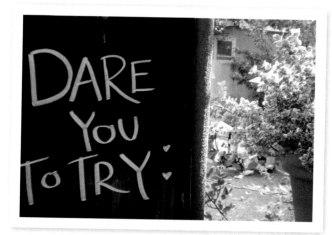

Not so crazy sexy Facts

We're in trouble like never before! If a decline in our well-being doesn't have anything to do with the crap we're shoveling into our mouths or breathing and walking through, I'll eat my cowboy boots (with Tabasco sauce). According to the World Health Organization:

- Cancer is a leading cause of death worldwide, and deaths are projected to increase by 45 percent from 2007 to 2030. New cases of cancer in the same period are estimated to jump from 11.3 million in 2007 to 15.5 million in 2030.

- In the United States heart disease is the number one killer. In 2005 more than 17 million people died of cardiovascular diseases such as heart attack or stroke.

Up to 80 percent of premature heart attacks and strokes are preventable with diet and lifestyles changes.

- More than 180 million people worldwide have Type 2 diabetes. Deaths from diabetes will increase by more than 50 percent in the next ten years without urgent action.

- Approximately 1.6 billion adults are overweight, and 400 million are obese. Globally, more than 20 million children under the age of five are overweight.

- In the 1970s autism affected about 1 in 10,000 children; today, in some states, it's 1 out of 150. Every twenty minutes, a child is diagnosed with autism.

BAD GENES versus BAD HABITS

The latest discoveries in genetic research are all the rage these days. Genes are touted as the miraculous great hope and the future of health and happiness. Science, medicine, and technology are all getting on the Gene Train. But when things go wrong with our health, genes often get all the blame. Whether it's cancer, alcoholism, cheating, or a fat ass, we're quick to pass the buck to our go-to scapegoat. As Dr. Dean Ornish suggested so eloquently in the foreword to this book, our genes are not our destiny. In fact, the relatively new science of epigenetics proves that our daily choices (diet, lifestyle, and environmental stressors) can actually change the way our genes express themselves—without changing our DNA. These non-genetic factors can literally switch disease, obesity, and other health issues on and off.

For example, only 5 to 10 percent of all cancers are caused by inherited genetic mutations, according to researchers at the Dana-Farber Cancer Institute in Boston. They, along with other top tacos, believe that between 70 and 80 percent of cancers are linked to diet and other behavioral factors like tobacco and alcohol—and not genetics. According to a 2009 study by the American Institute for Cancer Research, excess body fat alone causes more than 100,000 cancers every year. But here's the good news: If we can screw it up, then there's a good chance we can fix it, too. Nature meets nurture and beyond. Olé!

But not everyone agrees. After I gave a recent speech at a hospital in Georgia, a woman in the audience raised her hand to tell me I was wrong. In her mind, lifestyle choices didn't matter; if our name was in "God's book," we got sick. It's the book that matters, not the pepperoni pizza. I can't think of a

HOT crazysexy TIP

When you go veg the right way, you'll get all the nutrition you need from a varied plant-based diet loaded with vitamins, minerals, phytonutrients, oxygen, and enzymes. Don't believe me? Check out what the American Dietetic Association has to say: "Well-planned vegetarian diets are appropriate for individuals during all stages of the life cycle, including pregnancy, lactation, infancy, childhood, and adolescence, and for athletes. Vegetarians also appear to have lower cholesterol levels, lower blood pressure, and lower rates of hypertension and Type 2 diabetes than non-vegetarians. Furthermore, vegetarians tend to have a lower body mass index and lower overall cancer rates." The US Department of Agriculture (USDA) has some thoughts, too: "Vegetarian diets can meet all the recommendations for nutrients (including protein and calcium)."

more disempowered way to look at life. If that were the case, why bother trying to do anything other than pick lint out of your belly button? Didn't God give us free will? Isn't that the beauty and the bitch of being human?

Each of us has a genetic predisposition for something. Sometimes life flows by with no rough edges. George Burns lived to a hundred and certainly had a ball with his cigars, steaks, and highballs. He also had an incredible attitude ("Happiness is: A good martini, a good meal, a good cigar and a good woman . . . or a bad woman, depending on how much happiness you can stand.") that might have made up for the meat and martinis. The George Burnses of the world are very rare, however. Genes load the gun, but environment pulls the trigger. Think of it like seeds and soil. Without fertilizer, the seed can't always take root. You are the seed and your diet and lifestyle are the fertilizer.

This very important fact can freak a lot of folks out. Educating ourselves and taking charge of our health doesn't mean we're taking the blame. There's no need to point fingers or feel guilty. I'll never know what made me "sick." But it helps for me to ponder how I may have participated so that I can stop participating in my illness.

Next time you fill out your medical history, pause for a minute. Think about what runs in your family and also what's served on your family dinner table. A teacher of mine once gave me a helpful wisdom nugget. "Heart disease and diabetes don't run in my family," he said. "Sausages and doughnuts do!" It takes guts to look at the messy pain and truth in order to reevaluate the game you're running, but you can do it, sunshine!

BE A VEGGIE VIXEN

As Joni Mitchell, the high priestess of hippie, says, we've got to get ourselves back to the garden. Nature is the source of all things healthy; it is the ultimate surgical table and the basis of the Crazy Sexy Diet.

So what is this revolutionary game plan I'm gabbing about? Well, I gave you a snapshot earlier, but let's circle back. And don't worry, it's simple. You don't need a granola stigmata to figure it out. The Crazy Sexy Diet is a low-fat, vegetarian (or vegan) program that reduces inflammation and balances the pH of your gorgeous body with whole foods, low-glycemic fruits, raw veggies, alkalizing green drinks, and superpowered smoothies. On the CSD I encourage you to reduce or, better yet, eliminate all animal products, refined sugars and processed crap, and anything (other than an exotic vegetable) you can't pronounce. By decreasing the amount of acidic foods you eat, you give your body the chance to heal and repair naturally.

Your new mantra: Clean food in and waste out. An alkaline diet has the power to release stored

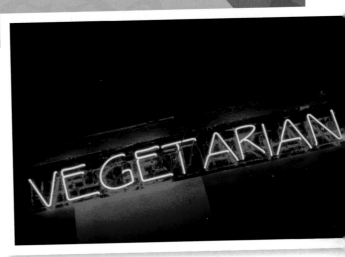

bullshit and toxins and truly set you free. As a result—and this is important—your pH comes into balance as does your overall health, your sinuses clear (and so do your zits), your taste buds resuscitate, your eyes sparkle, the dimples on your thighs will be gone (bye-bye!), sex will be better (ooohhh!), and so will your memory (especially good when you dig the person you have sex with), and your elimination system will work like a Ferrari (vroom!).

There's more, baby. When you understand why eating green and clean works at a cellular level, your enthusiasm for the Crazy Sexy Diet will grow like beans up a pole. Science is sexy and exciting! I'll explain why a plant-based diet is a great way to eat on so many levels—for health, bliss, beauty, even your purse. You may well lose fat on this diet, too, but that's just one of the fabulous side effects. Eventually you'll find your perfect fighting weight and forget about it because you'll be too busy enjoying newfound vitality and zest. That's because the Crazy Sexy Diet is not a temporary fix or a part-time hobby. It's a luscious lifestyle—a loss of dis-ease, a health gain program that is meant to last a long lifetime.

The Crazy Sexy Diet is a low-fat, vegetarian (or vegan) program that reduces inflammation and balances the pH of your dazzling body with lush whole foods, low-glycemic fruits, raw veggies, alkalizing green drinks, and superpowered smoothies.

WHY IT WORKS

By increasing the amount of raw and living foods and organic green juices and green smoothies in your diet while decreasing or (ideally) eliminating processed sugars, refined starches, animal products high in saturated fat, stimulants, and too much cooked food, you shift from an acidic interior environment to one that's alkaline- and oxygen-drenched. Yummy. This allows your magnificent body to recover from the constant barrage of stress and inflammation created by the Standard American Diet (aptly abbreviated as SAD) and lifestyle. Once your body repairs, it will renew. Eating this way is a miracle on your plate. The domino effect that occurs will influence every nook and cranny of your life.

Do you have to be a raw foodist to eat this way? Nope—steamed veggies that are crisp and crunchy

What you'll learn on the crazy sexy DIET

- The healing power of pH and how to eat alkaline foods in the right ratios.
- The importance of detoxification.
- How to keep your delicate internal ecosystem in balance.
- Anti-inflammatory raw foods = real energy.
- How juicing can change your life—make juice, not war.
- The benefits of going gluten-free.
- Why sugar is crack and how low-glycemic choices are a better option.
- The painful truth about meat and dairy.
- Stinkin' thinkin' and stress create acidity.
- Fun should be taken seriously.
- How to shake your ass . . .
- . . . and then place it on the meditation cushion.
- How to techno-detox.
- The importance of setting boundaries.
- Prayer and affirmations rule.
- You can do anything you set your mind to.

and lightly sautéed veggies count, too. How about a strict vegetarian or vegan? Nope and nope. The Crazy Sexy Diet is flexible. You'll enjoy healthier cooked food in smaller amounts. The acidic portions of your diet can include some animal products, but once you read how detrimental they can be to your health (and the planet), and how you don't really miss them, you may reconsider. And remember: Not all vegans are healthy. Even the most ethically conscious people can suffer from eating too many processed or overly acidic foods. French fries, Fritos, white bread and pasta, Pop-Tarts, Kool-Aid, Crisco, and many sugary treats are vegan, but they aren't exactly healthy. I call these misinformed veg-heads "muffin vegetarians." When I eat like a muffin vegetarian, I develop what is known as a "muffin top"—a puffy tube of blubber that hangs over my jeans. These well-meaning souls junk up on crap and excessive amounts of soy, and wonder why they're tired, fat, and sniffly. A vibrant and effective vegan or vegetarian diet means that the majority of your food is real and comes from . . . vegetables! (Duh.)

PICK A NUMBER— NOT JUST ANY NUMBER

The Crazy Sexy Diet has two levels: 60/40 and 80/20. I encourage you to aim for an 80/20 approach: 80 percent alkaline foods, 20 percent acidic. Though 80/20 is the goal, it's not the rule. For many people, especially those of you who are transitioning from the Standard American Diet, a 60/40 ratio is enough—and very healthy. Amen! The 60/40 ratio is a maintenance level, and if you're already in good health you will see amazing results by getting and hovering there. If you want to kick it up a notch or are recovering from an illness, an 80/20 (or more) ratio is your target. Touch it as often as you can. Start where you feel comfortable and stay where you feel the best.

Don't freak out at the math. I use the 60/40 or 80/20 ratios solely as a visual reminder. Look at your plate and divide it like a pie. More than half of the space should be taken up by fresh and organic delights from the garden. Make sense? Before we get to the heart of the plan, my posse of dynamic experts and I will teach you the whys and hows so that you can grab the steering wheel and zoom off on your own.

WHAT THE HELL HAPPENED?

Science and technology are totally groovy. Unfortunately, their misuse tends to complicate just about everything. A long time ago, in a galaxy far, far away, we ate real food! Getting a good meal on the table wasn't a multibillion-dollar industry driven by focus groups, slick advertisers, and government subsidies. Today chemical companies dominate the food business while their inbred cousins, the pharmaceuticals, are standing by ready to mop up the damage—and they're laughing all the way to the bank.

As my nerd crush, Michael Pollan, says in his must-read book *In Defense of Food,* "The chronic diseases that now kill most of us can be traced directly to the industrialization of our food; the rise

The Benefits of the
crazy sexy DIET

Okay, ladies, you've already heard about the vanishing cellulite and clear, sparkly eyes the Crazy Sexy Diet can bring you. Now see what you think of this list of further charmers. Your gal pals will beg you for your beauty secrets. Give them a high five and share your inner health regime—no sense in keeping something this great a secret.

- **A super-sexy glow**
- **Fewer colds**
- **Quick healing of both cuts and colds**
- **Terrific, regular, stink-free poops**
- **Healthy organs**
- **Clear skin and sinuses**
- **Leaner abs and a tighter butt**
- **A revved-up sex drive**
- **Better sleep**
- **Sweet breath**
- **Strong bones and pain-free joints**
- **Lower cholesterol and blood pressure (without pills)**
- **Balanced blood sugar**
- **Consistent energy**
- **Fewer blues, and more clarity**
- **Less "dis-ease"**

in highly processed foods and refined grains; the use of chemicals to raise plants and animals in huge monocultures; the superabundance of cheap calories of sugar and fat produced by modern agriculture; and the narrowing of the biological diversity of the human diet to a tiny handful of staple crops, notably wheat, corn, and soy. These changes have given us the western diet that we take for granted: lots of processed foods and meat, lots of added fat and sugar, lots of everything—except vegetables, fruits and whole grains."

OMG, he's red hot! And guess what? He's right. We no longer discuss actual food; instead we talk nutrients. Through the miracle of chemistry, we've lost sight of the forest for the trees, the kale for the vitamins. Tunnel-vision scientists assume it's the isolated elements in the kale that matter. But what if it's the glorious green leaf itself, in all its wondrous natural complexity, that rocks our world? What if we applied this dissection to people? If I cut myself into pieces and sold you my foot, would that help you navigate your journey better? We're greater than the sum of our parts, you, me, and the broccoli.

The truth is that real foods and fake foods will always be different—even if they have things in common on paper. Your body knows that a fresh tomato is better than corn syrup and red dye #40 ketchup; it also knows the difference between a sprouted whole grain and a partially hydrogenated hubcap with a hundred-year shelf life. But the food science game is about outdoing nature, and the rules say more is always better. If we find a good thing in the tomato, then we'll double it in the fake version. This hubcap has 11 grams of lycopene because our competitor has 10.

But how do we really know if these abstract ingredients actually work once they're isolated or created in a lab, then jammed into a noodle? They can glue some fiber to a jumbo sausage, but that doesn't make it good for you.

We've been brainwashed to believe that we no longer understand our bodies, that our innate wisdom is faulty or dangerous. And because it's all so confusing and scientific, we think we need a master's in nutrition just to get through dinner. But who has time for that? Enter the "experts." Don't ask where their research money comes from; just accept that they'll clear it all up with a trusty shopping list full of manufactured foods. Well, here we are with all this expert help and where has it gotten us? Broke, unhappy, dying early, and screwing up the planet on our way out the door.

Sadly, our government is a big part of the problem. Agencies like the Food and Drug Administration (FDA) and the USDA, which are meant to inform and protect us, often just increase our confusion. How? Because government food guidelines rarely mention food anymore! Instead we get gibberish about—you guessed it—nutrients. This is no accident. As family farms gave way to corporate consolidation over the past half century, our food system has been increasingly politicized.

A watershed moment that fueled the Age of Nutritionism came in the late 1970s when Congress, responding to growing awareness of the links between diet and disease, set out to rewrite the nation's health guidelines. Known as the McGovern Report, the new standards were clear in the first draft: Eat less meat and dairy. Sounds pretty straightforward to me, but the meat and dairy industries went bananas. Snap! Heads rolled and revisions were made. In the final draft this clear message had mutated into "reduce the amount of foods high in saturated fat." A generation later we're as lost and confused as ever. It shouldn't be so Zen koan complicated.

If products on the grocery shelves could speak, this is what you'd hear . . .

"Buy me, I have omega-3s!"

"Pick me! I'm doped up on antioxidants and have fewer calories than the fiberless bee-atch next to me. I mean, who does she think she is?"

"Oh yeah, well, I'm fortified with calcium and vitamin D. Plus, I reduce cholesterol and toe fungus!"

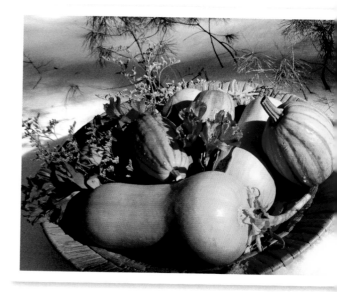

"Big whoop. I'm the new white meat, raised on a 'Happy Farm.' Sacrificing myself for your thighs was really fun!"

"Purchase me and you'll have more sex because you'll be skinnier and happier, and then you'll make more money and go to Paris and buy Gucci and meet Johnny Depp . . . and . . . and . . . [the package is thinking] . . . you'll solve global warming because I'm in a green box!"

The nonsense on packaging and advertising gets sillier all the time. The marketing behind a common breakfast drink claims that antioxidants found in this sugary, processed dairy mixture will strengthen the immune system. Well, a little understanding of that sexy science reveals that sugar and dairy actually suppress our immune system. Not to mention that any antioxidants in this pasteurized product are dead. No thanks!

Smart labels are another ridiculous campaign. Since when are Froot Loops healthy? Since never! Yet they have a smart label seal of approval. These mean absolutely nothing because there are no regulations or guidelines. The companies themselves determine whether or not a product is smart. And a lot of us dumbed-down consumers buy it hook, line, and sinker.

INNER AND OUTER GLOBAL WARMING

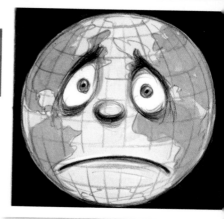

Wellness is not just about nutrition. It's also about ecology, spirit, passion, and culture. The Crazy Sexy Diet takes in all these interconnected issues. Illness made me look at myself in a new and honest way. It also woke me up to so many of the bigger issues facing us today. The choices we make really matter. What's happening in our bodies is a mirror of what's happening to the planet. It's our feeling of disconnectedness that keeps us from realizing we're all one organism.

Like the planet, our bodies have rivers, streams, lakes, oceans, soil, and air. These ecosystems make up our personal and planetary terrain. Both depend on a clean environment and a delicate balance. Chemicals poison our rivers and veins; pollution chokes our air and lungs; overacidity plunders minerals from our gardens and our tissues. pH affects everything from our forests to ocean life, bone strength, even cancer cells.

As we continue to expand our definition of wellness, we realize that the best place to find solutions to our personal and global challenges is on our dinner plates. Imagine the changes we could make if we simply started voting with our forks. One person can truly make a difference. You can start a revolution right at your kitchen table. In order to do that, let's touch upon some of the more immediate obstacles we face.

> **Imagine the changes we could make if we simply started voting with our forks.**

MONEY, TIME, AND FAMILY VIBES

Two common speed bumps to a healthier lifestyle are: "I can't afford it" and "I don't have time." Drive around them: In chapter 8, I'll give you lots of tips for cutting corners and stretching the dollar.

Yes, healthy food can seem more expensive, but if you choose wisely and buy in bulk, in season, and on sale, it's very affordable. In terms of dollars per nutrient, it's downright cheap compared with packaged food and animal products. It will certainly save you money in the long run. I'd much rather put my paycheck into my crisper than the medicine cabinet. My medicine cabinet is for emergency use only. In fact, there are only four things in it: Advil (for New Year's Day), Band-Aids, chemical-free tampons, and healthy cosmetics. Sadly, most Americans load those shelves with expensive "magic bullets." Your crisper holds the real medicine.

Check out yet another interesting fact from the sizzling Michael Pollan. He reports that in 1960, 18 percent of our national income was spent on food while 5 percent was spent on health care. Today 9 percent of our income is spent on food and 17 percent on health care. Clearly, the less we spend on food, the more we spend on health care. Take a look at your overall spending. I'll bet you can find places in your life where you can reallocate the do-re-mi. Do you really need more techno-crap? Shoes? Bags? Fashionable jeans? Even if you're not trying to find bliss with Blumarine, a realistic peek at your spending habits is in order. Your health deserves it.

As for time, I know you're very busy and the world demands a lot from you. But at the end of your life will you be bummed that you didn't plow through your master to-do list? Will you wish that you had worked longer hours and spent more time on Twitter? No way! You'll wish you climbed that mountain and took your kids to the moon. Astronauts like you need to be in good shape. If you don't make time to tune your instrument, then your music will always end on a flat note. And just like with money, I'll bet there are wasted minutes that could be better spent.

Weekends are a great time to catch up on meal planning. How about zone-out time? Exchange an hour of TV for washing, cutting, and bagging your veggies for the week and you'll save valuable time in the morning. Each day you commit to nourishing yourself will bring you one step closer to health. String the days together like pearls on a necklace.

Warning: A new you might freak some folks out. Family, friends, and food go together. If upgrading your diet stirs up a hornets' nest around the dinner table, step softly and use common sense. The best approach to a resistant loved one is blunt but polite honesty and leading by example. When your peeps see a happier, healthier you, they may follow in your footsteps. They should at least stop looking at you cross-eyed.

Others will want you to stay the same so they don't have to look at their own mess. Sorry! Change is frightening to those who find safety in routine. Plus, when you're living like you mean it, you're a force of nature. Now is the time to work on those boundaries and do what's best for you. It's not self-ish; it's self-*nurturing*.

PERFECTION AND BAR STOOLS

These changes may seem overwhelming at first. But this is not an all-or-nothing program. Most diets don't work because they don't take into account all the emotional work needed to stay on track. I've helped thousands of people transition to health, and what I've learned is that success has more to do

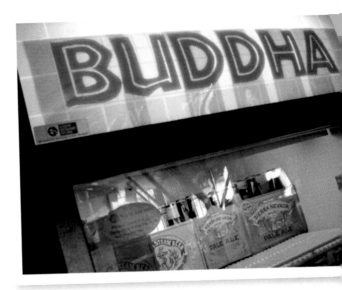

with being kind to yourself and dealing with your emotional shit than it does the food itself. If you stumble, cut yourself some slack!

Consistency is important, but you don't have to be perfect. Health is about keeping in an over-all "right" direction. Will you travel the same straight highway every day for the rest of your life? Snoozeville! You'll take scenic byways and even stop at honky-tonk bars. You may have a beer and chips in the afternoon followed by a shot of tequila for dessert. This is life—it's sweet, fun, and unpredictable. I am not perfect and I never will be. Perfect is beige. I am red hot! So are you. Red and Wild. You don't politely sit at tables—you dance on them. And after last call, you get back out on the health highway.

Why is it that so many of us make food so complicated and loaded? Food is nourishment; it's not the enemy. Food is romantic, creative, and divine. No diet that makes you feel deprived or socially isolated is worth it. I recognize that everyone is dealing with different circumstances, including our health, location, free time, income, family dynamic, and yes, our own psychology, to name a few. Do what you can and know that any change is better than nothing.

LET'S GO!

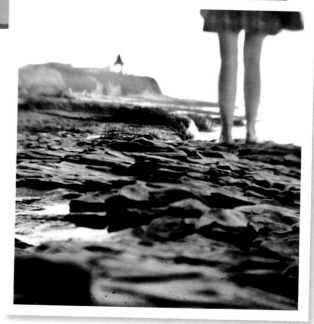

Are you ready to grab a bikini and dive in? Why wait till you're on the ropes to take charge of your well-being? It's gutsy to take a stand now! Devour the knowledge and dare yourself to step out of the comfort zone. Together we'll reset your dietary GPS and guide you to your dreams. Whether you're a CEO or a homemaker, life is complicated, gorgeous, staggering, and wild. Let your hair down and ride it bareback. Your new Crazy Sexy Diet helps you get over the finish line every single time.

Alysia Cotter Photography

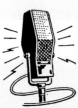

testimonial: Viki S.

I was diagnosed with rheumatoid arthritis eleven years ago and was put on several medications for it. The medications relieved the pain, but after being on them for several years I began to realize that all those drugs were not good for my body. I began to seek out sources for the new lifestyle I would need to pursue in order to achieve freedom from both the drugs and the arthritis and that's when I found Kris Carr and have been hooked on her ever since! Her energy, enthusiasm, and devotion to helping others are inspiring and her accessibility via her Web site (crazysexylife.com) is a true gift for those of us who are just starting to "lean into" a raw, vegetarian, or vegan lifestyle. After converting to an almost 100 percent vegetarian diet and incorporating yoga and acupuncture into my life as well, I have been off all of my RA meds for just over a year now!

CHAPTER 1 IN REVIEW

REMEMBER:

- You deserve to be healthy.

- The time to take charge of your wellness is now.

- Good nutrition will positively affect all areas of your life.

- The Crazy Sexy Diet is a low-fat, vegetarian program that emphasizes balancing the pH of your dazzling body with lush whole foods, low-glycemic fruits, raw veggies, alkalizing green drinks, and superpowered smoothies.

- Your grocery store can be your new pharmacy.

- Your daily choices can actually change the way your genes express themselves.

- The Crazy Sexy Diet is flexible—even small changes will give you great results.

- The CSD has two levels balancing alkaline foods with acidic foods: 60/40 and 80/20. Start where you feel comfortable and stay where you feel best.

- The CSD will teach you how to go vegetarian—and even vegan!—the right way, so you can get all the nutrition you need.

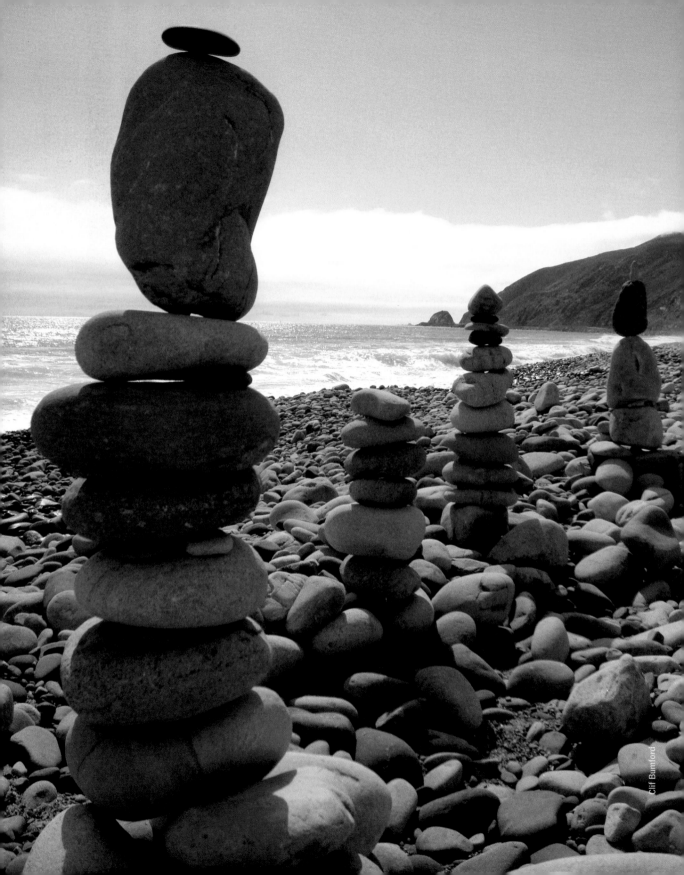

pHabulous

Have you ever been swept away by a toxic lover who sucked you dry? I have. Bad men used to light me up like a Christmas tree. If I had a choice between the rebel without a cause and a nice guy in a sweater and outdoorsy shoes, you can imagine who got my phone number.

Rebels and rogues are smooth (and somewhat untamed); they know the headwaiters at the best steak houses, ride fast European motorcycles, and start bar fights in your honor. In short, the rebel makes you feel really alive! It's all fun and games until he screws your best friend or embezzles your life's savings.

You may be asking yourself how my pathetic dating track record relates to your diet. Simple.

The acid–alkaline balance, which relates to the chemistry of your body's fluids and tissues as measured by pH. The rebel/rogue = acid. The nice solid guy = alkaline.

The solid guy gives you energy; he's reliable and trustworthy. The solid guy calls you back when he says he will. He helps you clean your garage and does yoga with you. He's even polite to your family no matter how whacked they are, and has the sexual stamina to rock your world.

While the rebel can help you let your hair down, too much rebel will sap your energy. In time, a steady rebellious diet burns you out. But when we're addicted to bad boys (junk food, fat, sugar, and booze), nice men (veggies and whole grains) seem boring. Give them a chance!

The cells of your body love the Alkaline Solid Guy, too. When your cells are at peace with their surrounding environment, they receive nourishment and release waste with ease. As a result, you experience a beautiful relationship with health. But when you eat, drink, think (and date) crap, your cells and inner environment become polluted.

The secret to super-sexy health is a slightly alkaline pH. It's that simple and that complex. Simple because the food you eat for optimum health is relatively accessible, inexpensive, and requires little preparation. Complex because we're all carrying around a lot of psychological food baggage that makes changing ingrained habits challenging.

Know this, sweetheart: Your diet and life-style choices will either help or harm your delicate pH balance and your overall health. In this chapter you learn how to groove in the optimum health zone. Grab the reins of alkalinity. Yee haw!

The secret to super-sexy health is a slightly alkaline pH.

pH Scale

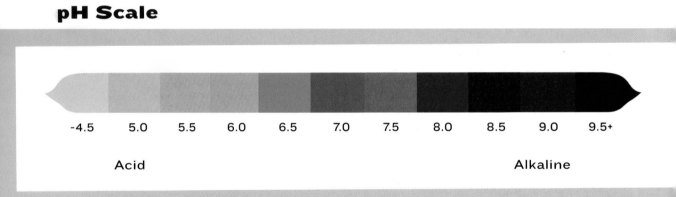

| -4.5 | 5.0 | 5.5 | 6.0 | 6.5 | 7.0 | 7.5 | 8.0 | 8.5 | 9.0 | 9.5+ |

Acid   Alkaline

pH 101

If you're like me, you ditched high school chemistry in favor of flirting and bumming cigs (acidic). Luckily, I went back to the books to learn what I missed. The pH of a substance tells you how acid or alkaline (basic) it is. pH is measured on a scale from 0 to 14. If something's neutral, it has a pH of 7.0. Above 7.0, it's alkaline; below 7.0, it's acidic. The higher above 7.0, the more alkaline it is and therefore the more oxygen it has; the farther below 7.0, the more acidic it is and the less oxygen it has.

Technically, *pH* stands for "potential of hydrogen." It is the measurement of hydrogen ions in a particular solution. The more ions, the more acidic the solution, and vice versa.

Okay, so why is this so important? Your brilliant body is designed to operate within a very narrow pH range. Optimally, you want to be a little on the alkaline side, with a blood pH of around 7.365. Blood is the most important, and therefore most protected, pH measurement. Even a minor fluctuation in your blood's pH (either too alkaline or too acidic) creates distress signals. Symptoms generally start out small and then ramp up as the imbalance continues.

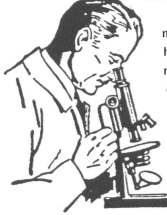

Everything from a runny nose to skin eruptions, heartburn, eczema, inflammation, arthritis, poor circulation, chronic fatigue, irritable bowel syndrome, a weakened immune system—even cancer— can be traced back in some way to an acidic inner terrain. In fact, a blood pH lower than 7.0 is extremely dangerous. Oxygen levels decrease, and cellular metabolism comes to a screeching halt. Guess what that means? Casket time!

It's much easier to become too acidic than too alkaline. Your body regularly deals with naturally occurring acids that are the by-products of respiration, metabolism, cellular breakdown, and exercise. But when our acidic diets and lifestyles add to the load, our bodies get overwhelmed. You can meet your amazing God pod halfway by shifting your pH balance toward the alkaline side. By simply eating a more alkaline diet—veggies, greens, fresh organic green juices and smoothies, sprouts, wheatgrass juice, certain grains, and other fabulous plant foods—you will explode with vibrant energy and well-being.

An acidic condition is also a breeding ground for bad bacteria, yeast, and fungi, while an alkaline environment helps keep these critters in check. We assume that colds and viruses happen when we "catch" a bug. In fact, many common infections are actually caused by bacteria that are part of the normal flora already present in our systems. When our diet and lifestyle choices suck, we create a fertile ground for them to multiply and revolt on the inside.

But it's not just diet that affects your pH. Lack of exercise, anger, drugs, cigs, and stress can all make you acidic. Stress is not a laughing matter or a badge of courage. The work-hard, play-hard, deal-with-it-later approach is a big pH no-no. Emotional stress releases acid-forming hormones such as cortisol and adrenaline that flood your system and muck up your soil. Plus, stress gives you wrinkles! When you're sixty you'll wish you had fixed that shit. Do the DIY now instead. Dump the doughnuts and chaos and watch the clock reverse.

PEE IS FOR pH

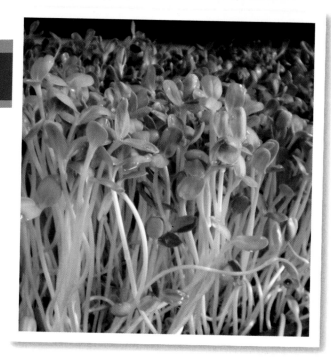

pH ranges vary slightly throughout your body. Your blood needs to be slightly alkaline for optimum health; so do your tissues. Your bowels, skin, and (for women) vagina should be slightly acidic—this helps keep unfriendly bacteria away. Your stomach is the most acidic environment in your body (with a pH that ranges from 1.6 to 2.4) due to the hydrochloric acid used to fight foreign invaders and break down foods, especially protein. Your saliva fluctuates the most but still should be slightly alkaline.

The simplest and most accurate way to read your pH is to test your urine—the most reliable bodily substance—with litmus paper strips, available online for about $10. They're similar to strips used to test chlorinated swimming pool water, so that you can do the backstroke without getting algae in your bikini. The litmus paper changes color when it's exposed to an acid or alkaline substance. The greater the color change, the more acid or alkaline the substance.

To test your urine, most manufacturers will tell you to simply hold the strip in the flow for a second or two and wait about ten seconds. Easy! Then just compare the color on the strip to the pH chart on or with the package. For optimum sparkle, your urine should fall in the 6.8 to 7.5 pH range. Keep in mind that the pH of urine varies, depending on what you eat and when. To get the best reading, blow off testing your first morning pee. Due to metabolic processes from the night before, it will generally be on the acidic side. If your first pee isn't acidic, it doesn't always mean you're in the zone. Quite the contrary, it could mean that you're not releasing acids the way you should. To get a more accurate reading, the best time to test your pH is on your second pee of the day and before meals or at least one to two hours after eating.

One reading of a test strip won't really tell you much, because levels fluctuate. It's best to track your readings a few times a day for a week or so to get a general idea of where you fall. Record your findings in a journal so that you can track your success. A few weeks of this will give you a pretty good snapshot of your body chemistry. As you transition to a more alkaline diet, you'll definitely see improvements. After a while you won't even need to test. You'll know exactly what will happen when you scarf hot wings and guzzle coffee.

It's important to keep in mind that pH operates on a logarithmic scale, meaning each increase of a single number in either direction away from 7 (neutral) is actually a multiple of ten. So when you move from 7 to 6 on the pH scale, that's ten times more acid; 7 to 5 is a hundred times more acidic; and so on. Coffee, for example, has a pH of around 4. Soda is a 2. Can you see why the SAD diet takes its toll? It's much easier on your bod to stay in an alkaline range than to try to restore it. In the blood it takes twenty times the amount of alkalinity to neutralize an acid. Sheesh, is it really worth that cup of Joe?

A few years ago I was teaching my husband about testing his pH and trying to encourage (force) him to eat more alkaline, raw foods and dump animal products completely. At the time, I was in my bash-people-over-the-head mode—and there is absolutely no worse way to approach the man I married. Several hours after he'd finished a burger, fries, and brews at our local joint, I asked him to test his urine. It was an 8, which is über-alkaline!

Naturally, I was shocked and began questioning all that I had learned. Then I hit the books to find out what was really going on. Animal products, fried foods, and alcohol are all highly acidic. In response, his cute bod was pillaging his mineral reserves. He was too alkaline because he had previously been too acidic—his body was overcompensating. Get it? A reading like this is a false positive. Once you understand the basics, you'll know when your body is truly in the zone.

ROBBING PETER to PAY PAUL

Ever hear the expression Something's got to give? Well, that something is gorgeous you! Your loyal and dedicated body will do anything it needs to do in order to keep you alive. It doesn't just "find" balance; it works dang hard to create it. If you've ever had a high fever, then you've experienced the desperation your body undergoes as it scrambles to regain control. A temperature of 98.6 degrees F is healthy, but 105—get your ass to the emergency room! On paper this doesn't seem like such a big number jump, but boy do those additional digits wreak havoc. Nausea, vomiting, chills, headaches, pain—these are just some of the symptoms felt as your body works to regulate your system.

Now imagine a similar cascade constantly taking place as your body tries to maintain proper pH. The Standard American Diet makes it very difficult to maintain a balanced pH. You eat the fiberless fried tushie with a side of coagulated mucus-creating moo juice (cheese), wash it down with a caffeine/booze fest, followed by a hunk of pancreas-smacking Sugar Snaps. You might love it going down, but your poor God pod is left to deal with the cleanup. One of the ways your body regains balance is by robbing from your precious mineral and enzyme reserves.

MINERALS AND pH

Your body needs super-sexy minerals in order to function properly. Since you can't make them, you gotta get minerals from your chow (preferably organic). In addition to the main minerals like calcium, magnesium, iron, potassium, and sodium, you need trace amounts of manganese, selenium, zinc, iodine, chromium, and copper. Your body uses these minerals to make proteins, enzymes, hormones, neurotransmitters, and everything else needed to tango.

So how do minerals affect pH? Foods rich in alkaline minerals, such as calcium, magnesium, and potassium, create alkalinity in the body, while foods containing acidic minerals, such as phosphorus and sulfur, lower the pH. A healthy diet stocks your body with plenty of alkaline minerals, while an overly acidic diet eventually maxes out the reserves. This forces your body to pull its own minerals to neutralize acids in order to keep your blood pH on the alkaline side.

One of the ways it does this is by mining alkaline minerals from your bones, teeth, tissues, and organs. When an alkaline and an acidic element hook up, they form a neutral salt. This salt no longer influences your pH (wow, chemistry is so titillating!). Think of this fabulous buffer system as your emergency stash of inner Tums. It's okay to use them occasionally, but not as a daily crutch. And if you don't replace your inner Tums with minerals from your chow, then the cabinet will be empty the next time you need it!

The major consequence of losing minerals from the body, especially teeth and bones, is osteoporosis and loss of bone density. One way that loss occurs—ironically—is by drinking too much milk. A high-protein, animal-based diet is extremely acidic. To compensate for that overload of acid, your body mines calcium from your bones and teeth to neutralize the acids created by the loads of milk you swill.

When the acid overload gets too high for your blood, your body dumps the acid out of your bloodstream and into your tissues. Next, your lymphatic system (the cleaning ladies of the body) tries to neutralize the acid and get rid of the waste. But the only way it can do that is to dump the acids back into your bloodstream. Can you spot the destructive cycle a mile away? And if your lymph system is already stuffed with acids, they start to build up in the tissues as well.

ENZYMES:
THE SEXY SPARK OF LIFE

Up to 95 percent of your body's activity is dependent on minerals, and one of their most important tasks is to help produce enzymes. Enzymes are little protein catalysts that ignite a gazillion complex and specific chemical reactions in the cells of every living plant or animal. There are thousands of different enzymes in your body, and they help with everything from digesting dinner to brain function to healing and detoxification. They're like the ultimate BFF, if you ask me.

You make two main types of enzymes: digestive and metabolic. Digestive enzymes break your food down into simpler, smaller bits that are easier for your body to absorb. The second you put grub in your mouth, digestion begins. It's a lovely step-by-step process involving your saliva, stomach, duodenum, pancreas, and small intestine.

Each of these fantastic organs secretes different enzymes at various stages along the way. Amylase in your saliva breaks down starch into sugar. In your stomach, enzymes like pepsin break down proteins. Lipase, an enzyme made in your pancreas and released into your small intestine, breaks down fats. If you lack adequate enzyme levels at any stage, food slips by and indigestion occurs. Add overeating and constant between-meal snacking and your body will have a hard time keeping up.

Here's another important factoid: Enzymes are both pH- and heat-sensitive. Cooking food above 118 degrees destroys enzymes. This doesn't mean that you can't eat cooked foods; it means that you shouldn't exclusively eat cooked foods. Highly refined and processed foods suck the most; they're completely devoid of enzymes (pasteurized stuff, too). Consequently, your body needs to make more digestive enzymes to get the job done.

But there's only so much energy to go around, so the more time your body spends making digestive enzymes, the less time it has to create metabolic enzymes. What are they? Metabolic enzymes basically run your body. They make every biochemical reaction in your 100 trillion cells possible. Metabolic enzymes build blood, tissues, and organs; repair your beautiful body; and help your cells produce energy and carry away waste. Obviously, these righteous little dudes are really important.

FOOD ENZYMES

There's one more important enzyme group to mention: food enzymes. For optimum health, we need to get additional enzymes from our food—especially as we age, because our bodies slow down enzyme production. Dang! Luckily, plant foods can supply the backup enzymes needed to keep us smart and sassy. Your body is a bank account, and food enzymes are the currency. Imagine making deposits instead of constant withdrawals. The more deposits you make, the more equity and interest you build.

By eating a vegetarian or vegan diet, with an emphasis on raw and living foods—which are loaded with their own enzymes—you give your body a break from the wear and tear of dining on too much cooked and acidic foods. The research of Dr. Edward Howell (often referred to as the father of enzymes) says, "Living organisms will secrete no more enzymes than are needed for digestion of a particular food." So when the foods you eat come to the party with the right amount of food enzymes, they don't drain the host. Instead, the enzymes in the food itself help the digestive

process; as a result, you use less of your own digestive enzymes.

If you're a curious dot connector, you may be wondering how pH-sensitive enzymes survive the tummy and its hydrochloric acid. This stumped me for years. Finally I came across a few respected sources that cleared this question up, including Dr. Gabriel Cousens, author of *Conscious Eating*. He offers evidence that there are actually two different sections of the stomach, the upper (cardiac section) and the lower (pyloric section). The upper section has a pH of about 5 to 6, which is important because food enzymes are still active in this range. Good news—grub stays in the upper section for up to sixty minutes, where food enzymes and enzymes from your saliva go to town. Once they hit the lower, more acidic section of the stomach, hydrochloric acid and pepsins take charge, especially on proteins, and food enzymes are only temporarily inactivated. Where does your chow go next? The alkaline small intestine—where food enzymes become active again in order to complete their

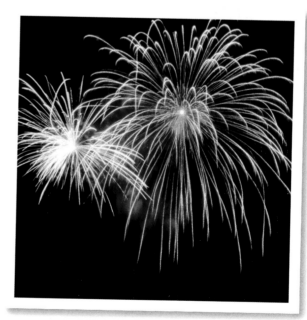

Tom Grundy

work. Food enzymes have another wonderful purpose: They allow your pancreas to take a break from secreting digestive enzymes. When this happens, your good old pancreas releases more metabolic enzymes for detoxification, renewal, repair, and general overall maintenance.

For all you pet lovers out there, food enzymes are an important thing to consider. Ever wonder why animals in the wild don't get the same chronic (human) diseases as our domesticated pets experience? The answer may lie in the power of enzymes. When animals are fed cooked, processed foods (sometimes filled with dangerous poisons from China), their bodies break down and they get sick.

In the early 1930s Dr. Francis Pottenger began a ten-year study involving more than 900 cats. He broke the cats into two groups. The first group was fed raw meat and raw (unpasteurized) milk. The second group was fed cooked meat and pasteurized milk. The cats on the raw diet remained disease-free and thrived. Over time, the cats on a 100 percent cooked food diet developed degenerative diseases, reproductive issues, and other health problems. Viva raw foods and enzymes for me, you, and Scooby-Doo.

THE POWER OF RAW AND LIVING FOODS

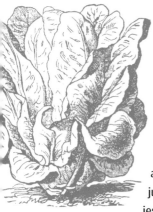

As you've probably guessed by now, whole and unprocessed raw and living foods add a huge amount of plant-based currency to your account. These foods are the fountain of youth. Leafy greens, wheatgrass, veggies, sprouts, certain fruits, nuts and seeds, grains, seaweeds, green juices, and smoothies flood our bodies with chlorophyll, enzymes, vitamins, minerals, phytonutrients, fiber, and oxygen. Happy, healthy cells love oxygen. They thrive on an alkaline, oxygen-rich, plant-based diet. Unhealthy cells (like cancer cells) or viruses, bacteria and other nasty microorganisms hate oxygen. They prefer an acidic diet high in animal products, processed and refined foods, and synthetic chemicals.

Ever hear of Dr. Otto Warburg? Well, he's sexy! And even though Warburg's been dead for decades, I still have a crush on him. In 1931 he won the Nobel Prize for his pivotal studies on the metabolism of cancer cells. His key revelation was that "Cancer has only one prime cause. It is the replacement of normal oxygen respiration of the body's cells by an anaerobic (oxygen deficient) cell respiration." In layman's terms, cancer cells are anaerobic, they thrive in an oxygen-depleted environment. Conversely, they cannot live in the oxygen-rich environment enjoyed by normal cells.

When we eat a plant-based diet, with an emphasis on raw foods, we assist our bodies in maintaining an alkaline (aerobic) environment. The more oxygen we get in our food, the more health we experience. Excessively acidic food creates an unhealthy cellular environment, which increases the chance of mutations. Raw and living foods (foods that are still growing, like sprouts) are the most alkaline, oxygen-rich foods we can eat. They're my prescription for optimum health. Because they haven't been cooked,

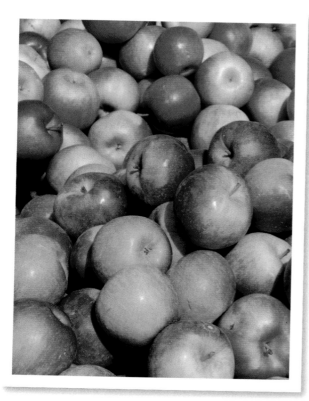

they still contain their life force. The fabulous fiber in raw food (or any fiber-rich food) also acts like an intestinal scrub brush, sweeping away debris. This allows your tubes to remain clear and ready to absorb nutrients from other healthy food. Your body loves all this life force, and so does your immune system!

In fact, your precious cells are like little batteries that run on energy provided the sun, either directly or indirectly. Directly: You eat the plant that grew in the sun that contains lots of vitamins, minerals, carbs, fat, and enzymes. Indirectly: You eat the vegetarian animal that ate the plant that grew in the sun and contains vitamins, minerals, carbs, fat, and enzymes. PS: Direct is best.

THE RAW LIVING REMEDY *with Dr. Brian Clement*

Your body is in great part H_2O (about 70 percent), otherwise known as water. A molecule of water has two hydrogen atoms and one oxygen atom. The hydrogen part is really important when it comes to making sure your bodily systems do not contain high acidity. This is a problem since the world of medicine estimates that approximately 60 percent of the global population does not consume enough of this essential nectar. To further complicate the issue, it seems that 40 percent of humanity lacks a little bell in the brain that tells them to drink. (Where did that go?)

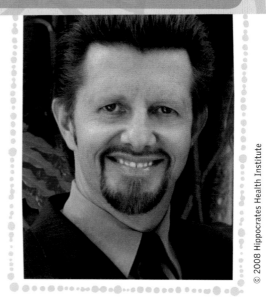

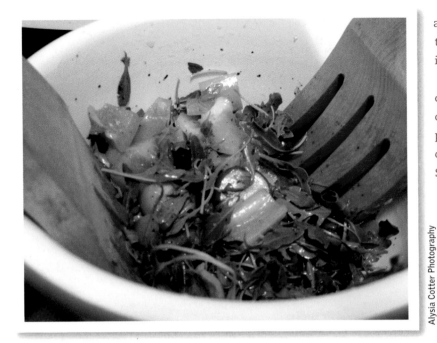

animal side, become a burden to the body, no longer supporting the metabolism.

Barbara Hendel, MD, a specialist in homeopathic medicine, says, "From a bio-physical perspective, food is a carrier of information to the body." She points out that you cannot grow an apple tree from cooked and processed apple butter, even if it is organic. Eating the apple raw gives you the bioelectrically charged nutrients that the human body thrives on. This choice of cuisine, which we have been feeding hundreds of thousands for more than half a century here at the Hippocrates Health Institute, has proven to be the nourishing healer that Hippocrates, the father of medicine, spoke about so eloquently.

Let's all come back down to earth: Eating raw organic, vegan, fresh food will bring your body what it needs to flourish, heal, and fight aging. The more you eat of this stuff, the less you have to worry about pH, getting old too soon, or lying in a hospital rather than enjoying wild romance with your favorite person.

Dr. Brian Clement, PhD, NMD, LN, and director of the Hippocrates Health Institute, is the author of several books, including *Living Foods for Optimum Health.*

When you consume adequate amounts of water, especially those pure and alkalized types, or raw juices, like watermelon juice on a hot day, your cells gulp it up. This hydration, in and of itself, is the greatest deterrent to a high-acid system.

Food is the second way we can regulate oxygen. Certainly the superstar bodybuilders are the organic vegetables. Germinated nuts, seeds, grains, and beans are the gold medalists. When eaten in their raw state, all these foods contain not only their inherent natural full spectrum of nutrients, but also water that contains hydrogen.

Yet even plant-based foods when processed and cooked, or fruit when harvested and eaten unripened, can all cause the bodies and bones to deteriorate. Some twenty years ago Dr. Theodore Baroody (author of *Alkalize or Die*) clearly stated, "The greatest nemeses to health are the tissue acids that have a difficult time leaving the body." Time and again research has demonstrated that processed foods, especially those from the

CHLOROPHYLL: LIQUID SUNSHINE

At the top of our supercharged alkaline health list is king chlorophyll. Think about it: Chlorophyll is what allows plants to absorb light from the sun and convert it into usable energy. Our very existence depends on the sun. We are interconnected to its energy on many levels, including what we shove in our mouths.

The chlorophyll in plants is what makes their leaves green and healthy. You can think of it as the blood of the plant—and in fact, it's similar to our blood. The difference is that the main atom in hemoglobin, the chemical that transports oxygen in your blood, is iron, while in chlorophyll it's magnesium.

Chlorophyll is a powerful blood builder. That's right, the blood of the plant literally helps heal and detoxify the blood of the body. It increases red blood cell production and enhances the cells' ability to carry oxygen. Chlorophyll strengthens the immune system, improves circulation, eases inflammation, and counteracts harmful free radicals. Foods especially high in chlorophyll are green (duh!), but if spinach is the only green food coming to mind, other concentrated sources are asparagus, green bell peppers, broccoli, green olives, kale, leeks, and turnip greens. By eating a diet high in chlorophyll, we dine on liquid oxygen, also known as sunlight—the very substance we need to stay alive and thrive.

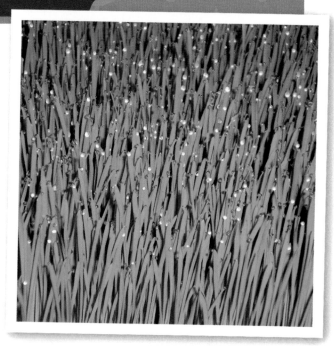

HOT crazysexy TIP

While eating raw fruits and veggies is optimal, quickly steaming, lightly sautéeing, or blanching food is the next best option, especially if you keep the inside of the plant crisp. For those with weak digestive systems, increasing your raw food consumption too fast can be ouchy on the belly. It's like expecting a couch potato to run a triathlon. Steaming and blanching helps break down the fibrous plant walls. As you heal your body, you'll be able to up the ante (and lower the heat).

FIGHT BACK AGAINST FREE RADICALS

Excess acid–forming foods put an enormous strain on the digestive system, liver, and kidneys. Neutralizing all that acid also creates extra molecules called free radicals, which damage our cells and rob electrons (life force) from healthy tissue. It's impossible to completely protect ourselves from free radicals (and we wouldn't want to). Some naturally form during normal metabolic function or as an immune response to stamp out bacteria and viruses. But too many free rads (from a shitty diet, carcinogens, environmental toxins, stress, etc.) up the ante on disease and premature aging.

What makes these molecules so dangerous? Basically, free radicals are molecules that have lost one of their electrons, and this makes them very unstable. Sort of how you feel when you can only find one of your Jimmy Choos. A free radical will latch onto any electron it can find. When these mini thieves steal an electron, that molecule in turn becomes a free radical, starting a cascade of them that can damage your cells. Take it from me—you can't trust too many free radicals. They talk a good game but they're moochers!

Your resourceful body produces antioxidant enzymes designed to quench the free radicals. This works because antioxidants are the givers. These generous little substances donate an extra electron to the greedy free radical. This stabilizes the little mutant and keeps it from bombarding other cells and snatching electrons from them. But if you have too many free radicals your body can't keep up. Downward health spiral, here you come!

One way to combat free radicals is to suck in less of the stuff that causes them in the first place. Another way is to give your body plenty of additional antioxidants found in (you guessed it) mostly raw, plant foods.

VITAMINS

Do you know why vitamins and minerals are always mentioned together? Well, like Bogie and Bacall, they're made for each other and need each other to be happy. A vitamin is an organic (carbon-containing) chemical compound that your body needs for normal functioning. Because your body can't make vitamins, you must get them from your food. There are thirteen vitamins in all, and you need tiny amounts of every one of them for good health.

Though vitamins are added to a lot of "fortified" foods, like breakfast cereal, bread, and OJ, it's not the same as consuming them in their natural form. Talk about backward: Manufacturers attempt to re-inject the nutrients they've processed out of natural foods, or add them to fake foods that never contained them in the first place. Synthetic laboratory vitamins are no match for the real deal. In some foods, vitamins and minerals are literally sprayed on! How dumb.

When you cook foods, you also reduce the vitamin and mineral value. You know those intoxicating stovetop smells? Well, suck them in, 'cause there goes a good portion of your vitamins and minerals. If you kill your broccoli, much of the vitamin C will end up in the cooking water, not in you.

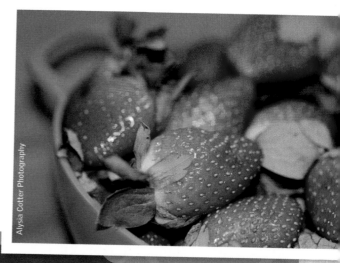

Alysia Cotter Photography

PHYTONUTRIENTS

Phytonutrients are like Secret Service agents that protect and fight off diseases in plants. Therefore, when you eat phytonutrient-packed plants, those little kickboxers help you fight free radicals and disease, too. Phytonutrients give plants their characteristic colors and flavors. Because they have at least one extra electron, phytonutrients are the ultimate givers. There are literally thousands of phytonutrients. But like enzymes, they are also heat-sensitive and are best eaten raw. Some researchers have found that cooking may help release certain antioxidants like beta-carotene and lycopene from plants' cells. But when you factor in the importance of retaining raw foods' powerful enzymes (and consider that they still contain butt-kicking levels of beta-carotene and lycopene in their raw form), it's still ideal to consume a mostly raw diet. Keep it real, keep it raw! Folks who get lots of phytonutrients in their diet tend to live longer, healthier lives.

Here's just a few of my fave phytos:

- **BETA-CAROTENE.** Found in orange-colored foods such carrots, sweet potatoes, and winter squash, beta-carotene is converted in your body into vitamin A. It's also found in dark green leafy vegetables, but the orange hue is hidden by our good friend chlorophyll.

- **LYCOPENE.** Found in tomatoes, watermelon, pink grapefruit, and some other foods, lycopene may help prevent prostate cancer.

- **LUTEIN AND ZEAXANTHIN.** Found in orange, red, and yellow foods such as corn, these phytonutrients help protect your eyes against age-related macular degeneration, the leading cause of blindness in older adults.

- **RESVERATROL.** Found in white, blue, and purple foods such as garlic, blueberries, grapes, and red wine, resveratrol is being studied for its life-extension possibilities. (Don't get too excited and run to the liquor store, sassy. Wine is still acidic, though it's a better choice than Red Bull and vodka!)

- **QUERCETIN.** Found in apples and onions, this may help prevent heart disease.

NOT ALL ACIDIC FOODS
ARE CREATED EQUAL

The problem isn't that we're eating acidic foods; the problem is that we are eating more acidic foods than alkaline foods. In the Standard American Diet, the typical ratio of acidic to alkaline foods is about 80/20—that is, 80 percent of the diet is acidic foods, while only 20 percent comes from alkaline foods like fresh raw vegetables. And we wonder why we have such a huge health crisis in our country?

We need to flip the ratio. Ideally, you want to have between 60 to 80 percent of your foods coming from the alkaline side—and only 20 to 40 percent coming from the acidic. But keep in mind that not all acidic foods are created equal. In fact, we need some acidic foods in order to get proper nutrition. For example, some nuts, grains, and beans are slightly acidic, but they're also protein powerhouses. Regularly including these gems in your diet is really important.

In his book *The Acid–Alkaline Diet for Optimum Health,* naturopath Christopher Vasey explains that the acids in plant foods are often referred to as weak acids. These acids include oxalic, pyruvic, citric, and acetylsalicylic. Animal proteins are called strong acids. These acids include, uric, sulfuric, and phosphoric. Neutralizing strong acids takes tons of energy and stresses your liver and kidneys. Since your kidneys can only eliminate a fixed amount of strong acids per day, the rest of the stuff is stored in your tissues. On the other hand, weak acids are easy-breezy to eliminate.

As Vasey suggests, there are no limits on the amount of weak acids that can be removed from your body by your cute kidneys. So as you can see, there is a huge difference between (slightly acidic) brown rice and (highly acidic) steak!

Even if you occasionally include a small amount of animal products in your diet, you'll be in much better shape than if you continue to stuff your face with them two or three times every day. No matter what pill, potion, surgery, or treatment our doctors come up with, if we don't participate in keeping our pH in balance, science and technology will forever remain a Band-Aid.

Remember, this is a direction, not a rigid absolute. Even though I have an exceptionally healthy diet, I still dip my vegan cupcake in a glass of champagne from time to time. The question is, how often? Regular bad habits deplete our core energy. Occasional compromises and tiny indulgences remind us that we're human. As long as the majority of the time you are giving your body what it needs (remember the bank account analogy), then the minor detours—when appropriate—actually help keep us on track. For a list of additional reading and wisdom feast your eyes on the crazy sexy resources in the back of the book.

A PEEK AT THE TOP ALKALINE FOODS

Here's a cheat sheet of yummy alky food and drink—have your fill!

Alkaline water.

Almonds, brazil nuts, sesame seeds, and flaxseeds.

Avocados.

Cold-pressed oils such as hemp, flax, and borage seed.

Moderate amounts of grains such as quinoa, wild rice, millet, amaranth, buckwheat. Exceptions: wheat, oats, and brown rice are mildly acidic.

Grasses, especially superpowered nutrient-packed wheatgrass.

Green drinks.

Green veggies—all kinds, but especially leafy green veggies such as kale, spinach, lettuces, collards, mustard greens, turnip greens, cabbage, and endive.

Lemons, limes, and grapefruits—although these fruits are acidic, they actually have an alkalizing affect in your body.

Lentils and other beans—in general, all legumes (beans and peas) are alkalizing.

Miso.

Oil-cured olives.

Raw tomatoes—but cooked tomatoes are acidic.

Root veggies, such as sweet potatoes, potatoes, turnips, jicama, daikon, and burdock.

Seaweed.

Sprouts!

Stevia (a sweetener).

THE ACIDIC RUNDOWN

Here's a list of some of the offenders on the 40/20 part of the CSD. Consuming them in moderation, limiting them to occasional indulgences, or eliminating them entirely is recommended.

Alcohol.

Animal protein: red meat, poultry, fish, eggs, milk, cheese, dairy products (these products are highly acidic).

Chemicals, drugs, cigs, heavy metals, pesticides, preservatives.

Coffee (even decaf), black tea.

Heavily processed foods, no matter what they are made of.

Honey, corn syrup, brown sugar, fructose.

Ketchup, mayonnaise, mustard (use sparingly).

Some legumes like chickpeas, black beans, and soybeans are slightly acidic but are valuable staples of a healthy diet.

Processed soy products tend to fall on the acidic side—enjoy them in moderation.

MSG.

Processed oils such as margarine, fake fats, trans fats, and refined vegetable oils.

Refined grains, wheat, and oats: White bread, pasta, and rice are highly acidic.

Soda, energy drinks, sport drinks.

Table salt (sea salt and kosher salt are better choices in moderation).

All salted and roasted nuts.

White sugar and sugar substitutes.

Yeast and vinegar (with the exception of raw apple cider vinegar).

Soy sauce (use sparingly and choose low-sodium tamari or gluten-free nama shoyu).

CHOOSING ALKALINE FOODS

How do we know if a food is alkaline or acid, and by how much? The most common method is to incinerate a sample of the food and analyze the mineral content of the ash. Not something you can do with a chemistry set from Toys "R" Us. At any rate, if the ash is high in alkaline minerals, the food will probably have an alkalizing effect. That's the theory, anyway. Because lab results and experts often disagree, the many books and Web sites that give alkaline and acidic food charts also disagree. Usually the disagreement is minor. In some cases, though, it's much bigger.

What I've done for this book is review all the reputable food pH sources I could find. I then applied my nutritional training to help me decide which sources were on the right track. Based on all that, I've come up with a mini sample alkaline/acid food list (see p. 35) to give you a basic idea of what foods to enjoy, moderate, or avoid altogether.

Whether a food is mildly alkalizing or mildly acidifying doesn't really matter very much. There are definitely shades of gray. What's far more important is for you to have a basic grasp of how all this works in order to make better choices.

HOT crazy sexy TIP

Love, laughter, and moderate exercise will help you maintain your acid–alkaline balance. Excessive GI Jane exercise is the opposite—it adds more acid to the body.

TOO-FRUITY!

Most fruits are slightly acidic (with the exception of avocados), because of their high fructose (sugar) content. However, in small quantities, fresh organic in-season fruits including all sorts of berries, apples, pears, grapefruit, and cantaloupe are fantastic. Think of a serving as one small to medium piece of "hand fruit" and 1 cup of berries or cut-up melon. Avoid canned and fermented fruits, preserves, jams, jellies, and processed or hybridized fruits that have lots of added sugar.

TAKE INVENTORY

So now that you know just enough about acid/alkaline foods and pH to make you dangerous, let's examine some of our favorite acid baths. Look at your plate, peek in your glass. What direction are you moving in? I don't know about you, but I used to make crappy meal choices three times a day, every day! Check out what my daily menu used to be (see sidebar):

An acidic menu like this makes you snooze, sneeze, swell up, gain weight, and get sick. These scraps are loaded with saturated fat and processed sugar, and they're desperately missing our pal fiber. In fact, every single food on this typical diet, with the exception of the broccoli (albeit dead), makes our bodies work triple time to counteract the cascade of chemical reactions coursing through us.

BREAKFAST: Coffee (with milk and Splenda), pasteurized OJ, some sort of fat-free, sugar-laden baked good, or fried eggs and bacon, toast with I Can't Believe It's Not Butter (well, what the hell is it then?).

11 A.M. CRASH: More coffee.

LUNCH: Hamburger (aka tushie) with a slab of individually wrapped and coagulated mucus (cheese), a white bun, fries, diet soda, and maybe a small salad (with a gallon of saturated fat – I mean ranch dressing).

4 P.M. CRASH: Coffee or diet soda and a pancreas-slapping candy bar.

DINNER: A mound of skinless baked chicken, macaroni and cheese, very boiled broccoli, and artificially sweetened and flavored iced tea.

DESSERT: One to ten cookies with shelf lives longer than me, or half a pint of low-fat frozen yogurt, followed by an emotional ass-whooping: "Why did I eat that? I sooo didn't need to eat that!"

DEBUNKING THE FAD DIET MYTHS

Now that I understand the importance of pH, I'm totally liberated from neurotic food calculations. Fad diets hold no power over me. When we consider the true measure of health, many popular diets just don't make sense. I don't need to know that I'm blood type O in order to shop for the right food for myself, and I certainly don't need a degree in anthropology. And while I appreciate the benefits of traditional diets, I stop at the emphatic advice to only eat foods from my culture of origin. I'm a Colombian, Irish, and Scottish mutt who respects and understands body chemistry. Empanadas, a slab of soda bread, and haggis (the boiled and minced windpipe, lungs, heart, and liver of a sheep) ain't gonna make me thrive.

Many nutritionists and wellness counselors advocate moderation without any true understanding of what that actually means. Moderation is not a green light. Moderation is education and conscious decision making. Will your body tell you what it needs? For sure! But will you be able to read the signs if you have no clue what to look for? My body used to tell me to eat two pints of Ben & Jerry's and flirt with cocaine. You can't be moderate if you don't know how to find your center. Once you build a solid home base, you can certainly play, stretch, and expand. But let's get our health ducks in a row first.

In the beginning of my journey with cancer I turned to a macrobiotic diet. In fact, during the filming of my documentary *Crazy Sexy Cancer*, macrobiotics was my sun, moon, and stars. The macrobiotic diet is a low-fat, high-fiber, predominantly vegetarian diet that is heavy on grains and soy products. After a while I felt depleted. Although I didn't realize it at the time, strict macrobiotic eating made me too acidic. This was my first clue that something was wrong.

Though there are many good principles to this way of eating, I was consuming far too much cooked foods and not enough raw, alkaline foods, water, and good oils—each of which I was prohibited from eating on the "healing" plan. I was told, "You're too yin, your cancer is yin, you can't eat raw yin foods." Try and explain that one to your oncologist!

Moving away from the macrobiotic diet was my first experience in "take the best and leave the rest." It got me off the horrible Standard American Diet way of eating, and for that I will forever be grateful. Plus, macrobiotics taught me how to tolerate seaweed, love kale, make healthy (and delish) soups, de-fart my beans, and use a pressure cooker without having to call 911.

When I did my first green juice fast (with lots of liquid nutrition), everything changed. Almost immediately my circulation came back and my blood work improved. With the addition of good fats, a moderate amount of whole grains, fresh veggies and low-glycemic fruits, my energy levels soared, my weight balanced out, and other chronic issues cleared up. From that day forward I was hooked on juice, adding more raw foods to my diet and recognizing the power of pH. Remember, raw foods isn't about eating only mangoes and bananas in 10-degree weather and then complaining about

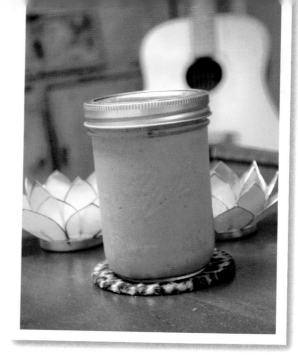

feeling drained. Leave that non-sense for the wacky fruitarians. Raw foods, Crazy Sexy style = more blood-sugar-stabilizing greens and less sugar, more chlorophyll and less chaos.

During the 21-Day Cleanse outlined in chapter 10, you will be flooding your body with alkalinity. This is an incredibly important component to the detoxification process, because the acids that have been stored in your tissue in order to protect the blood can finally be eliminated. With this new information, can you see why some of the popular cleanses can only take you so far?

If your body is a temple, then your mouth is the altar. From this day forward, vow to treat yourself like a Divine Being. Health is much simpler and far more scientific than we're led to believe. Your pH will never lie. That's why I honor and trust it. In return, it's given me phenomenal health in the midst of challenging circumstances.

You can't be moderate if you don't know how to find your center.

testimonial: Debbie Y.

Seven to ten years they gave me. No, not a prison sentence; it was my cancer prognosis. I was diagnosed with chronic lymphocytic leukemia at forty-seven, with a six-year-old daughter. I was to just watch and wait, no cure, no treatment, at least none that offered a longer life. The next six months I was adrift, lost in a sea of fear and hopelessness, searching for a way to heal, to live to see my daughter grow up. I read, I researched, looked for a ray of hope. Then I found *Crazy Sexy Cancer Tips*. I read it greedily and felt as if I had been airlifted to safety by Kris's wise words. Watch and wait meant seeing my white cells double in six months, a sign my disease was progressing. But now I had a life raft, a guide to living well and healing. The next five months were full of green juice, dry brushing, meditation, and a low-glycemic raw food diet. Then something magical happened, besides feeling incredible. My white count fell to half of what it was. I will always follow Kris's lead, for the rest of my long and healthy life.

CHAPTER 2 IN REVIEW

REMEMBER:

- Our bodies are designed to live within a narrow pH range—slightly on the alkaline side. Slip into acidity and a multitude of problems arise.

- Get curious about your pH—use urine strips to test and monitor it.

- Fight free radicals with healthy food enzymes, vitamins, minerals, and phytonutrients from raw, plant-based foods.

- Up your consumption of alkaline food, and reduce the amount of acid food you eat.

- Raw foods, Crazy Sexy style = more blood-sugar-stabilizing greens and less sugar, more chlorophyll and less chaos.

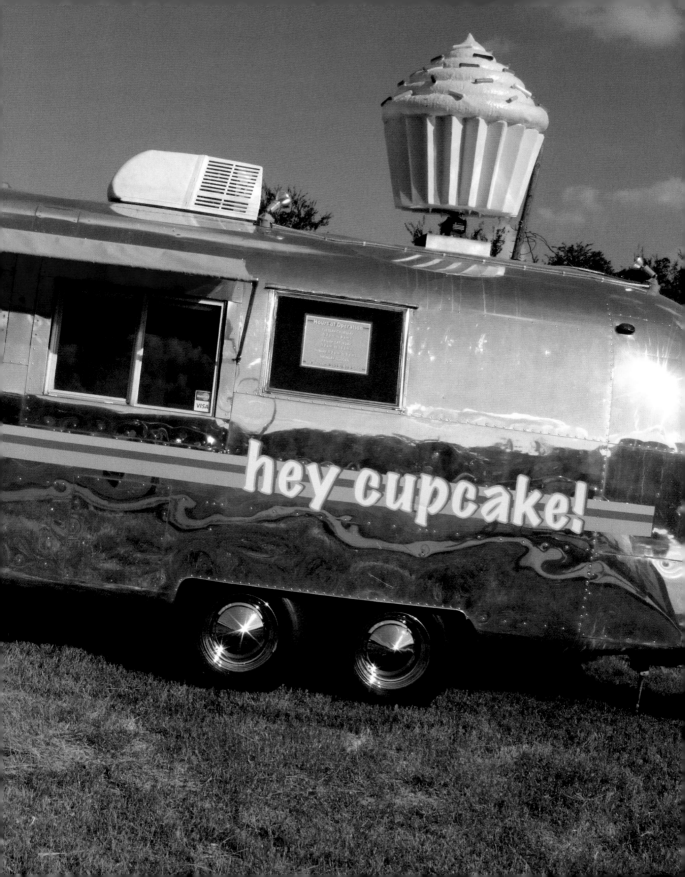

Cupcakes, COFFEE & COCKTAILS

Before we start our lesson on sugar and other stimulants, let's get one thing straight: You are sweet enough. You are sharp enough. Your natural, holy state is more than enough. You just think you need that extra boost. But your body knows exactly how to create it naturally. Keep it clean and lean. Dump the crack!

The real you knows exactly what I mean. In your original state you ooze magic honey. Unicorns want to lick you. Cupcakes and vodka just won't do. They distort your connection to your base energy. A bump, hit, sip, or snack will definitely make you soar for a hot mess of a minute. But like Icarus flying so high, the race to the sun will burn your wings and drop you on your fat, sugary ass!

Excess sugar (especially the devilish white stuff) robs your bod of minerals, lowers your precious pH, rots your teeth, wigs out your pancreas, feeds candida, fires up inflammation, osteoporosis, diabetes, and cancer, stresses your nervous system and adrenals, and screws with normal hormone function. It also makes you feel crappy after the initial jolt subsides. Sugar taxes your immune system and is highly addictive. Are some sugars better than others? Heck yeah, and you'll learn the best to choose. But in all cases moderation is key. Sweets are a treat, not an everyday event.

Look, I know firsthand how hard it is to heal addictions. I come from a scarf-and-barf, drink-too-much history. Date night with myself was a debaucherous romp into coma-ville. I'd buy a bunch of cookies and wine, pop the top button of my jeans, and chow down. Occasionally my higher self would guide me to the trash can before I finished every last crumb. An hour later my lower self would bark orders to pick through the trash and retrieve the delicious drugs like a back-alley junkie.

Elegant people don't dig through the trash. The chic and stylish don't attack their doughnuts with Windex. Yes, I admit it. The only way to keep my paws off the contraband was to blast it with Windex. Clearly, I was out of control.

Sugar taxes your immune system and is highly addictive.

SUGAR: THE LEGAL DRUG

Some of the most dangerous drugs are legal. And I'm not talking about the celebrity-killing pills; I'm talking about the narco-sweeteners that have overtaken the aisles of your grocery stores. Corporate yahoos do their best to greenwash and brainwash, but even the American Heart Association (AHA) is getting on board and imploring people to drastically reduce the amount of sugar they consume. In an article published in 2009 in the major medical journal *Circulation,* AHA researchers recommended that women limit their sugar intake to no more than 100 calories a day (about 6 teaspoons). For men, a limit of 150 calories per day (about 9 teaspoons) is suggested. That's way below the average of 355 calories (22 teaspoons) from sugar the average American consumes each day.

Still, even the low amount the AHA recommends is too much, in my opinion. Plus, do you know how hard it is to limit sugar when it's hidden in everything? You know that a 12-ounce can of cola has sugar in it—that's no secret (the equivalent of 10 teaspoons of sugar in the form of high-fructose corn syrup, or HFCS, in fact). Okay, but did you also know that HFCS is found in, well, many if not most packaged foods, including brands of applesauce, sushi, bread crumbs, baked beans, cough syrup, canned soups, and hundreds of other packaged products that have no real reason to include the sweet stuff? The US Department of Agriculture has estimated that we eat 79 pounds of corn sweetener per year. Not surprisingly, on average, a typical American consumes 150 pounds of sugar per year—and we don't even know it!

Manufacturers know that people like sugar, and they also know it is addictive. They play on the fact that sugar makes us feel better—temporarily—and that it's a comfort food. When you were a kid, were you ever bribed with cookies or candy? "If you're good and do such-and-such, you can have a tasty reward." Perhaps your BFF got dumped and desperately needed a shoulder to cry on. A perfect time for a "my condolences" pound cake! Or maybe, like me, you savored pound cake at funerals. Sugar is a delicious salve, and what used to be reserved for special occasions is now a 24/7 addiction.

Sugar makes us feel better for real reasons. It stimulates the release of dopamine (mood lube) in the brain. Naturally, when something makes us feel better, we crave more of it. It's a well-known fact that the cravings, withdrawal, and relapse symptoms of sugar addicts are similar to those of cocaine and heroin abusers. Their brains are actually wired in a similar way; yet another incentive for rethinking the sweet stuff bribery strategy. How about buying yourself a nice moisturizer when you're feeling low; or taking your kid to the movies or having a tickle fest, instead of indulging in candy when they've had a rough week at school?

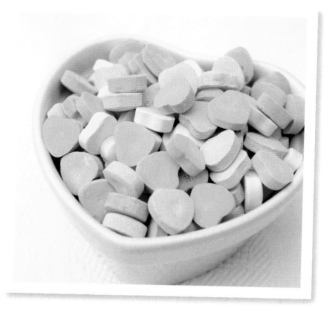

Now let's talk about my favorite organ, the liver. Excess sugar is stored in the liver as glycogen. Your liver is the cabinet and the glycogen is a stash of energy that your body can raid when it needs a boost between meals, during exercise, overnight, or while fasting. Like all storage spaces, however, there's only so much room. Someone who consistently overeats sugar and carbs will fill up all the storage space in the liver.

Once your liver is crammed full of glycogen, excess glucose is converted into fatty acids (triglycerides). It then enters the bloodstream and gets stored in your tissues. The good news: You don't have to rent a tire when tubing down the creek. The bad news: The tire permanently dangles around your middle. The really bad news: People who store more fat around their abdominal area are at higher risk for heart disease and diabetes. Are you picking up what I'm laying down? Too much sugar creates an unhealthy domino effect.

Before you graduate from my Prevention Is Hot cheerleading school, you really need to understand sugar at the physiological level. So let's get this party started with a basic tutorial.

CARBS 101

There's a lot of gabbing in the news about good carbs versus bad carbs—but what are they, exactly? First and foremost, carbohydrates are the starchy or sugary part of foods. When we think about sugar, naturally we imagine all things yummy and sweet. But in actuality, all carbs (including those that don't taste sweet, like pasta, bread, and potatoes) break down into glucose—the sugar your body uses for fuel. From your body's point of view, there's not much difference between a spoonful of sugar and a slice of white bread.

Carbohydrates come in two varieties, complex ("good" or "unrefined") and simple ("bad" or "refined"). Complex carbs such as whole grains, beans, and veggies are good for two reasons: First, they take longer to digest, therefore your blood sugar doesn't spike. This means your energy levels stay on a more even keel—no sugar highs and no crashes. No frantic search for guns, no scraping your torn self (in fishnets) off the concrete. Second, complex carbs come with a lot of other good stuff, like vitamins, minerals, enzymes, protein, and fiber. They fill you up and leave you satisfied.

Simple carbs often started out as complex, but they have a tragic fall-from-grace story. We humans tinkered with them. Once we started, we couldn't stop. In the process we refined, bleached, and blasted out all their goodness and starlight. What was once whole became a fake food in a deceptively perky package.

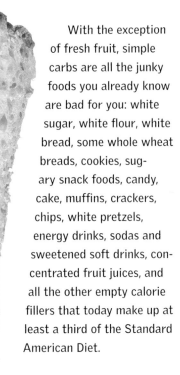

With the exception of fresh fruit, simple carbs are all the junky foods you already know are bad for you: white sugar, white flour, white bread, some whole wheat breads, cookies, sugary snack foods, candy, cake, muffins, crackers, chips, white pretzels, energy drinks, sodas and sweetened soft drinks, concentrated fruit juices, and all the other empty calorie fillers that today make up at least a third of the Standard American Diet.

Carbohydrates come in two varieties, complex ("good" or "unrefined") and simple ("bad" or "refined").

GLUCOSE

The fabulous Dr. Neal Barnard gives us a mini glucose lesson in chapter 4, but let's look at it here as it relates to our sugar tutorial. When glucose enters your bloodstream, your pancreas releases insulin, the master hormone of metabolism. Insulin has lots of jobs, but most importantly it regulates glucose levels by shuttling it to cells to use as fuel. But if a cell has all the fuel it needs for the moment, insulin carries off the extra glucose to be stored as fat. So far, so good—because everyone needs a little cushion for the pushin'. However, a diet high in simple sugar and refined carbs dumps a ton of glucose into your blood very quickly. As a result, your pancreas is forced to barf out additional insulin, which isn't good for you or your pancreas.

This is one vicious cycle. Over time you may develop insulin resistance, which makes your body less effective at regulating blood sugar. Insulin resistance also affects your ability to use stored fat as energy. In other words, you can't lose weight as easily when there's a bunch of insulin coursing through your body. But it's not just about weight. Too much glucose and insulin is a major culprit in many diseases.

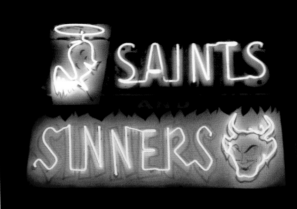

SUGAR AND CANCER

Now, I don't want to vilify sugar (glucose) here, because it's the fuel that feeds all our cells, healthy or unhealthy. Everything we eat gets broken down into glucose eventually—even fats and proteins if needed. In fact, without glucose we couldn't survive. However, if you have cancer—in any form—it's best to avoid all refined sugars and carbohydrates and cut back on high-glycemic fruits. Why? Read on, studious vixen!

One of the reasons cancer cells are so freaky is that they are extremely hungry. Their metabolism is much higher than that of healthy, normal cells. Yet cancer cells are totally inefficient. They have to work much harder and burn more glucose to produce the same amount of energy as healthy aerobic cells. It's sorta like comparing a Prius (healthy cells) with a gas-guzzling SUV (cancer cells).

But cancer cells are crafty, too. To obtain the amount of fuel they need, cancer cells have around nineteen times more glucose receptors than normal cells. This allows them to come to the party first and suck up the fuel fast. One of the ways that cancer cells process their fuel is through fermentation, which converts sugar to energy without using oxygen. Remember our little pH lesson? Healthy cells love oxygen; cancer cells don't. Their clunky anaerobic metabolism produces a lot less energy. So to stay alive, cancer cells need a bigger fuel supply. What's the best way to get quick fuel? Sugars and carbs!

If you have any doubt about sugar and cancer, consider how a PET scan works. Patients are injected with a tiny amount of radioactive glucose (sugar). The test measures the parts of the body that absorb the most glucose. Greedy cancer cells light up like fireworks.

But it doesn't stop there, and as you just learned, you can't talk about glucose without mentioning insulin. As David Servan-Schreiber, MD, writes in his book, *Anticancer: A New Way of Life,* "The secretion of insulin is accompanied by another molecule, called IGF (Insulin-like Growth Factor), whose role is to stimulate cell growth. Furthermore, insulin and IGF have another effect in common: They promote the factors of inflammation that also stimulate cell growth and act as fertilizer for tumors." Bottom line: Excess insulin in the body tells cancer cells to grow, baby, grow.

Need I say more? That's all I need to know as a cancer patient. And though some well-respected experts disagree, I'm not taking any chances! Whether we're talking normal cells or cancer cells, the cycle is the same: The more sugar you eat, the more acidic (anaerobic) you become, the more you tax your immune system, the more stress and inflammation you create, the more insulin and IGF circulate in your body—and thus the more opportunity for cancer cells to grow and divide.

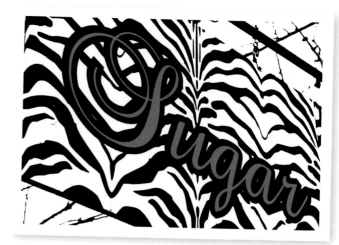

THE GLYCEMIC INDEX

How can you learn to make better choices when eating carbs and sugar? Enter the dazzling glycemic index (GI), a measure of how quickly and how high a particular carbohydrate raises your blood sugar level. GI is a numerical ranking system that compares a given food to a pure sugar, such as white sugar. Because white sugar is all carbohydrate, it's designated 100 on a scale of 0 to 100. The GI is a measure of carbs only; fats and proteins have no effect on the score.

Foods with a high GI value are almost always refined, simple carbs. Conversely, foods with low GI values tend to be unrefined, complex carbs. The difference between high- and low-GI foods lies mostly in how much fiber they contain. Fiber slows the digestion of sugars and keeps you even and peaceful. That's why a plant-based, low-GI diet is one of the central tenets of the Crazy Sexy lifestyle.

Familiarize yourself with the glycemic index—it's a terrific tool. As a rule of thumb, any food that has a GI rank below 60 is a good choice, especially if you need to watch your blood sugar. In fact, people who stick to a low-GI diet are less likely to develop diabetes and other medical life lemons. And guess what? Not only can low GI diets prevent nasty diseases, they can also help to reverse them. Amen, glitter explosion!

I've listed the GI Index of many common foods. Keep in mind that the index measures grams of carbs, not grams of food. In other words, it doesn't tell you how much you have to eat to get that gram. For example, a big bowl of beans might contain the same quantity of carbs as a small bowl of fruit. If you want to learn more, *The GI Handbook* by Barbara Ravage and *The New Glucose Revolution* by Jennie Brand-Miller and Kaye Foster-Powell are both great books for self-study.

GLYCEMIC INDEX VALUES
OF SOME COMMON FOODS

BEANS	GI VALUE (per gram of carb)
Black beans	30
Black-eyed peas	42
Chickpeas	28
Kidney beans	28
Lentils (red)	26
Lima beans	32
Mung beans	39
Soy beans	18
Split peas	25

FRUIT	GI VALUE
Apple	38
Apricot	57
Apricot (dried)	30
Banana	52
Blueberries	53
Cantaloupe	65
Cherries	63
Grapefruit	25
Grapes	53
Kiwi fruit	53
Mango	51
Orange	42
Papaya	59
Peach	42
Pear	38
Pineapple	59
Plum	39
Raisins	64
Strawberries	40
Watermelon	76

VEGETABLES	GI VALUE
Carrots	47
Corn	48
Green peas	45
Baked potato	85
Sweet potato	59

note: Most vegetables are 0 on the GI index, including broccoli, cabbage, cauliflower, cucumber, green beans, chard, kale, lettuce and other salad greens, and spinach.

GRAINS	GI VALUE
Barley	25
Buckwheat	54
Bulgur	48
Cornmeal	68
Millet	71
Quinoa	53
Rice (brown)	48
Rice (jasmine)	109
Rice (white)	56
Wild rice	57

SOURCE: Jennie Brand-Miller and Kaye Foster-Powell, *The New Glucose Revolution*

ARTIFICIAL SWEETENERS ARE NOT *sexy*

Only a few decades ago, plain old sugar was about the only game in town to satisfy a sweet tooth. But as Old Cane started to get a bad rap, the chemical companies began cranking out one artificial sweetener after another. Dr. Ginger Southall of the Hippocrates Health Institute emphatically states that the use of chemical sweeteners of any kind—aspartame, NutraSweet, Equal, Sweet'N Low, saccharin, Canderel, and even Splenda—is not advised, tootsie. "Artificial sweeteners are potent nerve toxins and never should have been approved as safe for human consumption. They have the potential to freak out and damage your nervous system—your brain and nerves—leading to a variety of symptoms from migraine headaches to unexplained seizures, dizziness, depression, and vision problems. They are even linked to cancer, obesity, and diabetes. I bet you didn't realize how many of these human-made tasty toxins you gobble up on a daily basis. They hide out in thousands of your favorite foods, including diet meals, flavored waters, popular drink mixes such as Crystal Light, many commercial

HOT crazy*sexy* TIP

Read the label for what the manufacturer says is a serving size. The label can claim a product is low in sugar, but the portion size might be unrealistically small—two tiny cookies, for instance, out of a pack of ten tiny cookies.

salad dressings, and—ready for this?—even over-the-counter medicines like Alka-Seltzer, tooth-pastes, gum, vitamins, and those Listerine breath strips! Even the stuff that 'tastes like sugar because it's made from sugar' is highly processed and has been laced with chlorine." Yum!

So what are the sweeteners of choice on the crazy sexy diet? Raw organic agave, yacón, and, even better, stevia are great choices. Pick them up at the local health food store or even at the good old standard supermarket.

CONTROLLING CRAVINGS

When I first started on my Crazy Sexy Diet, my cravings didn't care one bit that I was trying to get healthy—my body was used to crap and wanted more. Before sundown I was an alkaline angel, but when night fell I'd hear that eerie spaghetti-western music in my head. You know, the tune that plays when the white-powder outlaw rides into town. I'd slam the door, roll the armoire

in front of the windows, and grab my handy sawed-off shotgun.

Useless! The fudge brownies (à la mode) would find their way to my lips. Once down the hatch they created a wild (yet numbing) effect that made me want to move to a brothel! The only way for me to break the pattern was to acknowledge and then grin and bear the craving cyclone until it passed.

Here are a few effective ways to ride the wave of the crave without falling into the ocean:

- Have a snack that's high in protein and some fat, such as nuts, seeds, and avocado.

- Sip a hot herbal tea with a bit of agave or stevia.

- Get a satisfying boost from a zesty lemonade made with a couple of freshly squeezed lemons, stevia, and mint (or strawberry).

- Juice up a nutrient-packed green drink or smoothie with some good fat in it, like coconut or avocado.

- Enjoy a rice cake with almond butter or a baked sweet potato.

- Go for a small piece (about 1 inch square) of dark chocolate—75 percent or higher cacao is best. Cacao rocks; carob, too. Savor them slowly.

- Sip some almond milk with cocoa and stevia.

- Snack on a cup full of low-glycemic fruit salad (pears, apples, blackberries).

- Grab a piece of wood and bite hard like a Civil War amputee.

- Floss, brush, and gargle with natural minty mouthwash. It sends the signal that the office of eating is temporarily closed for business.

- Change your environment until the crisis passes. Go for a walk, call a friend, take a bubble bath, cuddle your pet, have hot sex!

SNEAKY SUGAR

Think those cookies sweetened with concentrated fruit juice instead of white sugar are somehow "healthier"? Isn't brown sugar better than white? Nope. Sugar is sugar, no matter what alias it hides under. Ditto for labels that claim "no sugar added" or "contains only natural sugars." Those are often weasel words used to trick you. If you spot any of these words on the ingredients list, the product contains sugar:

Brown sugar
Corn sweetener
Corn syrup
Corn syrup solids
Dextrose
Fructose
Fruit juice concentrate
Glucose
High-fructose corn syrup (HFCS)
Honey
Invert sugar
Lactose
Maltose
Malt
Malt syrup
Maple sugar
Maple syrup
Molasses
Raw sugar
Sucrose (table sugar)
Sweetened carob powder
Turbinado

INFLAMMATION with Lilli B. Link, MD

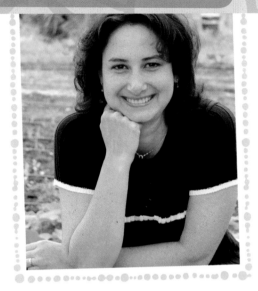

By the time I completed medical school and residency, these were a few of the things I had been taught:

- Inflammation plays a role in only a few chronic diseases.

- Diet is important in heart disease and diabetes, but otherwise doesn't make much of a difference.

I've since learned that inflammation has a role in cancer, heart disease, diabetes, inflammatory bowel disease, asthma, Alzheimer's disease, high blood pressure, and on and on. As a matter of fact, I wouldn't be surprised if every chronic disease has some inflammatory component. Now, you might be wondering if that is good news or bad news. I think it's good news because it means there is something you can do about it: Eat an anti-inflammatory diet.

You may be familiar with the throbbing feeling you get after a paper cut, or the warm, red swelling that comes with a sprained ankle. These are the white blood cells and other molecules that come along to attack and destroy the cells causing the problem and then clean up the debris. But sometimes this process goes awry.

To describe it simply, if the wrong signals are sent to your immune system, perhaps by eating inflammatory foods, the inflammatory cells and other molecules may mistakenly get called into action and instructed to attack healthy parts of your body. The more time they spend in circulation—because you're eating inflammatory food throughout the day, for example—the more opportunity they have to damage your blood vessels and lead to a heart attack, or destroy

cartilage and cause rheumatoid arthritis, or alter DNA and change healthy cells into cancerous cells.

An easy way to control this activity is to add more anti-inflammatory foods to your diet. The first three foods on the list are vegetables, vegetables, vegetables! For anyone who disregards dietary recommendations because they are always changing, remember this: No one ever said, "Don't eat your vegetables!" They are healthy in so many ways, including the fact that they decrease inflammation. Veggie sprouts are great, too. Ounce for ounce, they are even healthier than the full-grown vegetable. And you can grow them on your kitchen counter.

Fruits also have a wonderful array of nutrients and are anti-inflammatory. They get second billing because some are really sweet, like dates and tropical fruits. Go for the fruits with the least natural sugar, such as strawberries, blueberries, raspberries, apples, and grapefruit.

One of the most talked-about components of an anti-inflammatory diet is omega-3 fatty acids. These are healthy fats and one reason fish gets promoted so heavily. In fact, cold-water fish are full of omega-3s, but they are also often full of toxins such as mercury from the waters they live in. There are a number of vegan options for omega-3 fatty acids, like algae (I know, not everyone is going to think this is vegan or even sounds appealing). Nuts and nut oils are in general anti-inflammatory because of their high omega-3 content. Flaxseeds and oil, hemp seeds and oil, chia seeds, walnuts, and marine phytoplankton are all high in omega-3. Extra-virgin olive oil is anti-inflammatory, too, probably because it is high in monounsaturated fatty acids such as oleic acid.

Spices such as turmeric (the ingredient in curry powder that makes it yellow), ginger, and hot red peppers are anti-inflammatory, as is garlic—so don't be afraid to flavor your food! One last anti-inflammatory food to mention is green tea, which is great in moderation.

Now on to inflammatory foods. I'll start with sugar. In medical school I was thrilled to learn that, unless you had diabetes, the only problem with sugar was that it caused cavities. Ah, if that were only true! In a 2004 study of patients with diabetes that appeared in the journal *Metabolism*, participants were given a sugar drink, and then their blood was tested for inflammation.

Within one hour of drinking the sugar, the level of inflammation in their bodies rose, and the effect lasted three hours. You can just imagine what might happen if you are snacking on sweetened foods throughout the day for months on end.

Refined grains come next as an inflammatory food because, once they are digested, they are almost the same as sugar. When you eat a piece of white bread or white rice, the food turns into blood sugar so quickly, the effect on your body isn't much different from eating sugar itself.

Trans fats are also among the worst inflammatory offenders. These fats are created when vegetable oil has been partially hydrogenated to become solid at room temperature, like stick margarine.

Heating food to high temperatures is also pro-inflammatory. A 2002 study in the journal *PNAS* looked at two groups of people with diabetes. One group was fed food heated at a low temperature; this decreased the amount of inflammation in their bodies. The other group was fed the same exact food, but heated to a high temperature; this increased the amount of inflammation in their bodies. So even if you are not eating a raw vegan diet, at least try not to grill, roast, or fry your food. Instead, simmer, steam, or gently sauté food over medium to low heat. Use a slow cooker to cook dried beans. You are better off cooking something

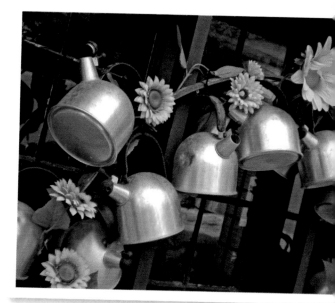

at a low temperature for a long time than at a high temperature for a short time.

Being overweight is inflammatory. Fat cells, especially the ones that sit around your waist and belly, are the most dangerous because they actually produce inflammation. Keeping your weight in check is a great anti-inflammatory move—and an anti-inflammatory diet will help you do that, including the Crazy Sexy Diet.

Lilli B. Link, MD, is a board-certified internist currently practicing as a nutritional counselor in New York City. She specializes in raw foods and integrative nutrition. Visit her at www .llinkmd.com.

GLUTEN-FREE LIVING

While we're talking about sugar, carbs, and inflammation, let's talk about a major health issue that is often overlooked: gluten intolerance. It's a pain-in-the-ass condition that could easily be affecting you. In fact, if you've tried everything, been tested for everything, changed your diet significantly, and still feel lousy, then avoiding gluten might be the missing link to your vibrant health. Sensitivity to gluten—a protein found in wheat, rye, and barley—could be the culprit behind digestive problems like bloating, cramps, diarrhea, fatigue, achy joints, and even skin rashes. People who are more than just mildly sensitive to gluten have these symptoms big time. They have celiac disease, which can cause severe damage to the small intestine and serious nutrition issues.

Remember what Dr. Link just taught us about what happens in our bodies when we eat inflammatory foods? Well, an allergy to gluten is similar. It's like having an inner injury created by a foreign invader. What happens next? Your awesome body goes into whoop-ass mode to destroy the bad guy (gluten). Unfortunately, this heroic gesture only causes more inflammation. Ugh, I'm exhausted.

A surprisingly large number of people are sensitive to gluten and experience some or all of the symptoms whenever they eat wheat and the other grains. But since most people don't know about the effects of gluten sensitivity, they chalk their symptoms up to other problems such as irritable bowel syndrome or even depression and then pop medications that don't really help, when all they really need to do is change their diet.

Celiac disease used to be thought of as a rare childhood phenomenon. It turns out that it's much more common and doesn't always start in childhood. More than two million people in the United States have celiac disease—that's 1 in every 133 people, and the number could actually be as high as 1 in every 100 people. According to researchers at the Mayo Clinic, for every person diagnosed with celiac disease, it's possible that there are as many as thirty more who have it but haven't been diagnosed. They say celiac disease is four times more common now in the US than it was in the 1950s.

There's a simple way to know if gluten is not your friend: Stop eating it and see how you feel. It's amazing how chronic problems, like fatigue, bloating, gas, and diarrhea, clear up when you kick out the gluten.

Gluten intolerance or celiac disease could be the culprit lurking behind any of these symptoms:

Diarrhea, especially if it happens often for no apparent reason

Abdominal pain

Bloating and gas

Foul-smelling poop

Anemia

Depression

Irritability

Joint pain

Mouth sores

Muscle cramps

Skin rash

Osteoporosis

Neuropathy (tingling or pain in the legs and feet)

The only treatment for gluten intolerance or celiac disease is a gluten-free diet. Gluten is found in every single form of wheat. That includes durum (the kind used for flour), semolina (the kind used for pasta), spelt, kamut, einkorn, farro, and other forms of wheat, such as wheat germ and bulgur. Gluten is also found in grains related to wheat: rye, barley, and triticale (a cross between wheat and rye). If you have celiac disease, you have to completely eliminate these grains from your diet and your life.

If you're sensitive to gluten but don't have celiac disease, it's possible that you can eat small amounts of gluten-containing grains. The degree of gluten sensitivity varies from person to person. Wheat has the most gluten, so you probably want to stay away from it completely, but you might be able to have small amounts of rye and barley.

Avoiding gluten completely isn't easy. It means never eating wheat bread, pasta, cereal, and almost all processed foods. That's because processed foods often have hidden gluten in the form of food additives, preservatives, and stabilizers. Frozen french fries, for instance, often have added gluten. There's even gluten in lipstick.

Life without pasta? No way! Just choose gluten-free brands—there are lots of delish kinds to select from. You can also eat grains, such as brown rice, wild rice, amaranth, corn, buckwheat, millet, teff, and quinoa. Some people can eat oats without any problems, although others may have to skip them because oats are often processed in the same plants where wheat is processed, and cross-contamination may occur. Check out glutenfreeoats.com for more information. Instead of wheat flour, you can use gluten-free flours made from a variety of grains, legumes, nuts, and seeds. In fact, many supermarkets today have a good selection of gluten-free breads and other products, and it's amazing what great gluten-free stuff you can get online. And don't forget that fruits, veggies, leafies, beans, potatoes, squashes, seeds, and nuts don't have gluten, so you have tons of great options.

GO GLUTEN-FREE with Mark Hyman, MD

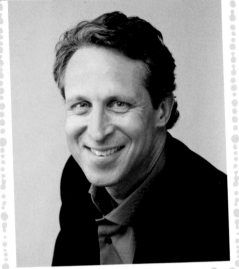

A recent large study in the *Journal of the American Medical Association* found that people with diagnosed, undiagnosed, and "latent" celiac disease or gluten sensitivity had a higher risk of death, mostly from heart disease and cancer. The findings were dramatic. There was a 39 percent increased risk of death in those with celiac disease, 72 percent increased risk in those with gut inflammation related to gluten, and 35 percent increased risk in those with gluten sensitivity but no celiac disease.

This groundbreaking—and startling—research proves you don't have to have full-blown celiac disease to experience serious health problems and complications—even accelerated death— from eating gluten. Yet an estimated 99 percent of people who have a problem with eating gluten don't even know it. They ascribe their ill health or symptoms to something else.

A review paper in *The New England Journal of Medicine* listed fifty-five "diseases" that can be caused by eating gluten. These include osteoporosis, irritable bowel disease, inflammatory bowel disease, anemia, cancer, fatigue, and canker sores, as well as rheumatoid arthritis, lupus, multiple sclerosis, and almost all other autoimmune diseases. Gluten is also linked to many psychiatric and neurological diseases, including anxiety, depression, schizophrenia, dementia, migraines, epilepsy, and neuropathy (nerve damage). It has also been linked to autism.

Of course, that doesn't mean that all cases of these conditions are caused by gluten intolerance—but if you have a chronic illness, you may want to follow an elimination/reintegration diet. While a blood test can help identify gluten sensitivity, the only way you will know if this is really a problem for you is to eliminate all gluten for a short period of time (two to four weeks) and see how you feel. Check the labels of all foods. They must indicate, by law, the potential presence of wheat, peanuts, and soy.

For this test to work, you must eliminate 100 percent of the gluten from your diet—no exceptions, no hidden gluten, and not a single crumb of bread. If at the end of the test period you feel great, ditch the gluten. If you go back to gluten and feel at all bad, you know you need to stay off gluten permanently. We do not need gluten to live; it is completely optional as far as our health goes.

If you are still interested in knowing more, gluten allergy/celiac disease tests are available through Labcorp or Quest Diagnostics. They help identify various forms of allergy or sensitivity to gluten or wheat by looking for various antibodies that signal gluten-related conditions. You can also have an intestinal biopsy, although it is rarely needed if gluten antibodies are positive.

When you see your test results, consider that I believe any elevation of antibodies is significant and worthy of a trial of gluten elimination. Many doctors consider elevated anti-gliadin antibodies in the absence of a positive intestinal biopsy showing damage to be "false positives." That means the test looks positive but really isn't significant. We can no longer say that. Positive is positive and, as with all illness, there is a continuum of disease, from mild gluten sensitivity to full-blown celiac disease.

Mark Hyman, MD, author of the best-selling *The UltraMind Solution* and other books, is a practicing physician and a pioneer in the emerging field of functional medicine, which strives to use new research to understand and treat the underlying causes of disease.

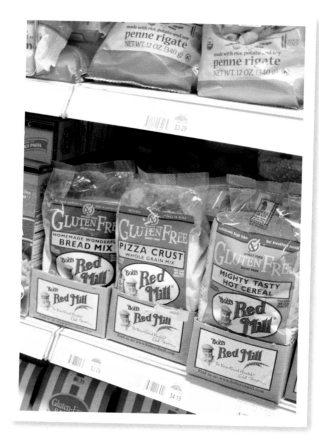

SOCIAL LUBRICANTS AND JAVA

Now for the liquid lovers. And who doesn't love a cup o' Joe and a glass of red? Enjoy them from time to time; just don't make them an everyday habit. Like sugar, these mischievous Casanovas are highly addictive. Once you dip your toe in, they've got ya. Your adrenals, kidneys, skin, breath, cholesterol, blood, and blood pressure will thank you when you dial down your consumption.

Coffee is extremely acidic and causes considerable dehydration. Remember that minerals are required to balance pH. Kiss these minerals goodbye as you piss them down the toilet along with

your hot cup of Starbucks. Those who advocate regular moderate use claim that coffee contains beneficial properties. Maybe so, but that doesn't take into account the whole picture. We can't dissect the good from the bad in order to make the case for our health choices.

In addition to being acidic, coffee beans are roasted. These beans have oils in them. Roasted oils become rancid and clog up your lovely liver. It's kinda obvious that this stuff isn't good for you. The fact that you get the jitters when you drink it, and migraines when you don't, should tell

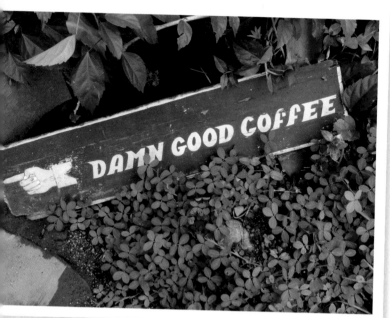

caffeinated drinks. See your gynecologist if you ever feel even the slightest lump. If it turns out to be a benign cyst, you may want to check out evening primrose and vitamin E. (I myself take about 1,000 mg of evening primrose and 400 to 800 IUs of vitamin E.) This helps tremendously; within a few weeks the cysts will likely disappear.

GETTING OFF THE JOE

Getting off coffee isn't all that hard, but don't do it cold tofurkey. If you're a heavy caffeine consumer, dumping it suddenly might make you a homicidal zombie. Wean yourself slowly over a week or so.

- **MAKE—AND DOWN—A GREEN JUICE!** The more juice you drink, the fewer outside stimulants you'll need. Green juice, a mixture of glorious green veggies and herbs, is loaded with a hefty blast of sustainable energy.

- **HAVE A CUPPA GREEN TEA,** white tea, or yerba maté. The relatively small amount of caffeine in these drinks will definitely help you transition. Bancha and genmaicha teas both have a very earthy taste and are made from older green tea leaves picked at the end of the season. Kukicha, made from the twigs, stalks, and stems of the tea plant, contains the tiniest amount of caffeine. Kukicha tea has a slightly alkalizing effect and is good for bellyaches.

- **TRY CACAO (RAW CHOCOLATE),** the coffee alternative that will knock your socks off. It contains only trace amounts of caffeine. I love making a superfood smoothie out of cacao, nut milk, stevia or agave, and vanilla—add a few goji berries and a banana. Or try making a delish hot chocolate by heating some hemp milk and adding a scoop of cacao and a dash of agave!

you something. How about insomnia? Coffee is definitely the enemy of restful sleep. And if you're dealing with anxiety, panic disorders, or a really stressful job, coffee will only exacerbate the chaos. If a cold sweat really turns you on, then by all means, drink up.

For those gals looking to start a family, a 2008 study in the *American Journal of Obstetrics and Gynecology* found that mamas who guzzled high doses of caffeine during pregnancy (around 200 milligrams or more per day, or two cups of brewed coffee) had a greater risk of miscarriage than those who drank less caffeine; the more caffeine the women drank over 200 mg, the greater their risk of miscarriage. Think about it: Who wants to live in a house that's dirty and stressful? The baby's immature metabolism hits the roof while your coffee break strangles the blood flow to the placenta. And that includes sodas with caffeine, energy drinks, and black tea.

Women who are prone to breast cysts will also want to stay away from coffee and other highly

- **BREW UP SOME TEECCINO** with almond or hemp milk and a drizzle of agave for an amazing cup of herbal coffee. Teeccino is made from grains and doesn't contain any caffeine. It does have a wee bit of gluten in it, so if you're sensitive you may want to avoid it.

- **SAMPLE CHICORY,** a totally natural product made from a perennial plant. It's completely caffeine-free and can be brewed right in your home coffeemaker (after you give it a good washin'). Use 2 to 3 tablespoons of ground roast chicory for each cup of brew desired. Vary the amount to suit your taste. Sweeten with hemp or almond milk and a drop of stevia.

- **IF THERE'S NO WAY IN HELL YOU'LL TRY ANY OF THESE** alternatives, then at the very least choose organic, shade-grown coffee and cut back to no more than one cup per day. Remember, flirt—don't marry! Some folks do the half-caf, half-decaf thing, or transition to decaf. Find companies that use a water process to strip the caffeine. Most store decaf brands use toxic chemicals that often remain in the brew. And buy the best you can afford—if you're going to drink coffee, it might as well taste good.

BUT JESUS DRANK WINE!

Guess what? You ain't Jesus. Now, I'm not saying you have to haul your ass to AA and sober up ASAP; breaking (gluten-free) bread and sipping vino is a lovely thing. Let's just make sure we're keeping it in a healthy range. Like coffee, alcohol is very acidic. Even when consumed in moderation, alcohol interferes with your ability to absorb nutrients. So let's define moderation: That's one drink daily for women, and no more than two drinks a day for men. What's a drink? One 12-ounce serving of beer, or one 5-ounce glass of wine, or 1.5 ounces of 80-proof distilled spirits. I bet some of y'all thought moderate was a 7-Eleven Big Gulp with a phat blast of Jack. Nope!

More than two drinks a day increases your risk of liver disease, high blood pressure, and cancer. For women, the risk of breast cancer goes up the more you drink—women who regularly have more than two drinks a day are at higher risk than women who drink less or don't drink at all. Since alcohol creates blood sugar spikes, people with diabetes need to be particularly careful—their levels can peak and plummet into a dangerously hypoglycemic range.

If you're trying to lose weight, alcohol will sabotage your plans. Drinking too much booze messes with your ability to know if you're full. Since alcohol contains tons of empty calories, overdoing the sauce will make you look like a bloated hag. Excess booze also damages your cute little intestinal villi and reduces the absorption of nutrients—especially folate, vitamin B_{12}, and calcium. Though some studies suggest that moderate amounts of red wine (one glass daily) have health benefits, especially to the heart, these perks can be obtained in other ways that are far less risky. Fresh-squeezed Concord grape juice, anyone?

The problem for most overworked folks is that alcohol can easily become the go-to chill outlet. I sure as heck love my Zinfandel unwind. But I'll also admit that sometimes I find reasons to drink or look forward to drinking. When alcohol (or drugs) are your primary tool for stress reduction or coping in public situations (aka social lubricant), it's time to assess the situation. An occasional spirit might just be the thing you need to lift your spirits—but occasional doesn't mean every day.

If you turn into someone else when you suck it back—big red flag. I once dated a dude who had a history of alcohol abuse in his family. Though he didn't drink on a regular basis, he still had a drinking problem, because when he did get lit, he changed. One night he changed too much, but that's a story for another book.

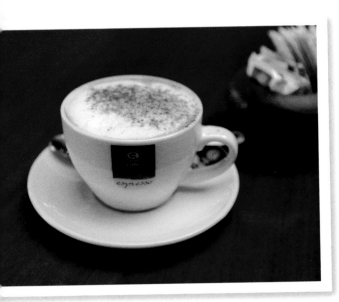

It's scary to put our acidic vices (sugar, booze, coffee, pills) on the back burner for a while. But there's no need to stress out over the idea that this is "forever." The clean, real you is "for now" and if she feels good, then visit her often. You won't turn into a boring wallflower if you clean up your night-club act. Listen to your body and ease up. If you perceive this way of eating and living as depriva-tion, then your cravings will skyrocket. That's why it's important to address all the stinkin' thinkin' in our hearts and heads as we clean up our terrain.

Plan your blow-its. Mini splurges in small propor-tions won't tip the health cart over completely. You can still meet your friends for a latte or a glass of organic wine (invite me!). As long as you stay in the 60/40 to 80/20 ranges, the majority of the time, your body will get the boost it needs to shine on, you Crazy Sexy diamond.

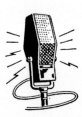

testimonial: Lauren L.

I have Crohn's disease and have been on medications for four years. I had been eating well for over a year but was still on prednisone and unhappy about it. Then I found Kris. I jumped right into her Crazy Sexy Diet! When I started her program I was feeling sick, tired, and just plain terrible from the high dose of prednisone. Who would have known that in just twenty-plus days I would be off the prednisone and feeling better than ever? Cutting gluten out of my diet, juicing, green smoothies, and eating mostly raw foods have helped me to feel incredible. While I am not cured yet, I still have hope and I know that with this diet, being cured is within reach. The CSD has brought my clarity to a new level. I have more energy than I've had in a long time and I am full of light.

CHAPTER 3 IN REVIEW

REMEMBER:

- Get the sugar out—too much (and not even that much) of this habit-forming substance wreaks havoc on your blood sugar levels, mood, and weight. That goes for the artificial stuff, too.

- Simple carbs like white bread and pasta, pastries, and potatoes are basically sugar in disguise.

- Choose most of your food from the low end of the glycemic index scale.

- Consider going gluten-free for a while to see if you feel better—if you do, can the wheat products.

- Buzz off—cut down on or eliminate caffeine and alcohol.

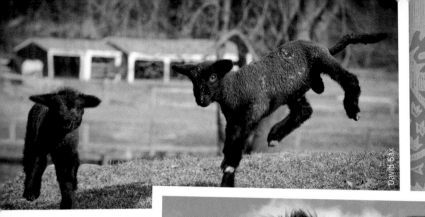

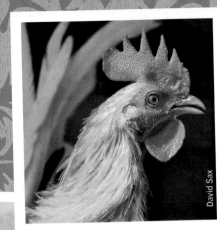

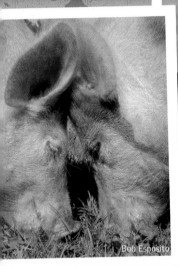

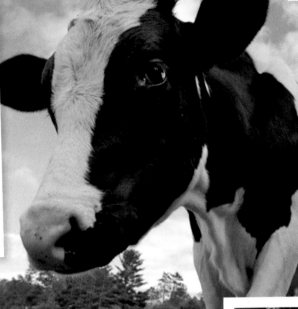

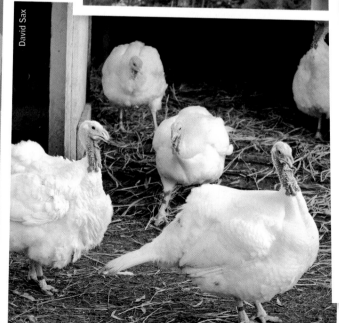

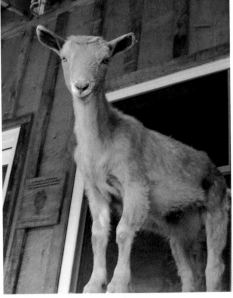

TUSHIE &
MILK MUSTACHES

Are you ready for the Crazy Sexy Truth about meat and dairy? Of course you are! You're a fearless Wellness Warrior full of rebellion and fire. So with that in mind, it's party time and I'm gonna give you a big, phat prezzie. In fact, this treasure is so top-shelf that it'll keep you young, cute, and alive! Going veg is one of the best decisions you can make for your health and the planet. Period. Your organs, blood, bones, teeth, and private parts will thank you. Private parts? Yes, sassy, I'm talking sex drive! There's no better way to light the night than to eat right.

I meant it when I said in chapter 1 that any change in your diet is a good one—a change from the SAD to an increase of plant-based foods is

something I'll celebrate along with you. But I won't lie: For optimal health we need to reduce or, better yet, dump animal products. We're just consuming too much of the stuff and it's making us sick. It's that simple, kitten, and I'm going to try some tough, straight talk to help you to think of meat and dairy in a new way. This is the talk that I got that helped me change my life. Maybe it will help you too. If not, I still love you.

There's a lot for you to digest in this chapter, and you should take some time (and enzymes) to do so. My goal isn't to convert you to veganism or judge and criticize you if you eat meat. My goal is to share the tools, knowledge, and facts I've learned so that you can have the best day, week, month, life ever! If at the end of this chapter your eyes are more open and you make healthier, cleaner, and more conscious animal product choices, then I've done my job. The day we stop questioning is the day we stop learning. Question where your food comes from and you'll be in much better shape. What matters most is your longevity, so take the best, leave the rest, and fasten your seat belt, doll!

If your meals consistently revolve around corpse multiple times daily, you might become one sooner than you planned. I imagine that this statement is quite unsettling for some—it sure was for me. I grew up across the street from a small, family-owned dairy farm. Shooting milk from the udder straight into my mouth was fun. Udders also made terrific weapons. Point, aim, squeeze, and if you got lucky you'd nail a passing farmhand. (I adored causing trouble. It wasn't till I tried my first bit of Red Man chewing tobacco that those sneaky bastards got me back. "You can swallow it, tastes like candy." After about thirty seconds I barfed on his boot and cried. Touché.)

At home our daily meals revolved around animal products, and the options were either decadent or gross. My fiery Colombian grandma was a very imaginative chef who loved buckets of butter, Julia Child, and anything she could flambé (that is, douse with booze and set on fire, including, on occasion, the curtains). On decadent days dinner would consist of coq au vin or curried chicken. On gross days we might get tongue, chipped beef on toast (which has an uncanny resemblance to vomit), and Spam cake sandwiches. What's a Spam cake sandwich, you ask? Alternating layers of the mysterious meat and slices of white bread covered with cream cheese. Since presentation was everything, Grandma topped the Spam cake with colorful cream cheese flowers made with food dye and

shot through a pastry-decorating bag. Sometimes the cakes would even have my name on them.

Grandma loved to experiment. The day my mom went into labor with me, she had just finished a big bowl of kidney stew with red wine glaze and scalloped potatoes. I imagine that the little me said, "Enough is enough, I'm outta here, lady!" My tastes, on the other hand, were simple. I could live happily on the following five foods in rotation: hamburgers, cereal, Ritz crackers with Cheez Whiz, PB&J, and fries.

When I was ten years old, I learned that there was a God, because she had finally answered my prayers by opening a Burger King on Route 22. I immediately begged Grandma to take me, but since fast food was foreign she vetoed the request in her thick Colombian accent. No (in any language) is not a word I stomach well—never have, never will. Though I didn't have wheels, I still had my feet. So I pillaged her coat pockets and took off on a 10-mile walkabout. Boy, were those fries worth the hell I caught. In one fell swoop, I tasted freedom, independence, theft, and trans-fat-drenched carbohydrates. I was hooked. For the next two decades, fast food would be my rebellious comfort.

So I'm not just blowin' smoke up your ass, I understand how hard it can be to change patterns. I found this amazing lifestyle because I was on the ropes. While I loved animals and nature, I didn't make the connection. A burger has a face and is unhealthy? When we shake it up and wake it up, we realize that ignorance isn't yummy or sexy or responsible.

Do you have to change everything all at once? No! As I said at the start, I don't expect you to go full-tilt boogie. Even if you don't eliminate flesh completely, cut way back—snip snip, trim trim. The American Dietetic Association recommends that meat, poultry, and fish portions should be no more than the size of a deck of playing cards—about 3 to 4 ounces. Even for Texans!

To help you avoid (or at least reduce) animal products, let me clarify what we're talking about here. Meat = a being with ideas, a mother, family, and community. Dairy = liquid meat from the breast of an animal with ideas, a mother, family, and community. I know it seems pretty obvious, but I come across a lot of folks who need a little "what's a sentient being" refresher because they're under the false impression that chicken and fish don't count.

The vast majority of our animal consumption comes from the famous five: cow, chicken, turkey, pig, fish. But there's a whole Noah's ark of notable noshables: lamb, goat, duck, bunnies, frogs, buffalo, deer, elk, ostrich, shellfish, snakes, eel, monkey, and for all you Deliverance guys still out there, squirrel. Basically, if it moves, we find ways to kill it and eat it. Then there's milk. Cow, goat, and sheep are our main sources for cottage cheese, cream cheese, cheese, sour cream, butter, ice cream, yogurt. And what about eggs? Somewhere along the line we mistakenly grouped them with dairy (probably because they're next to butter and cheese in the grocery store), but actually they are considered meat since they contain similar nutrients—and because they're little chicken fetuses. So as you upgrade your diet, keep these critters and critter products in mind.

Here's an easy way to reframe your plate. Think of meat and milk products as the supporting cast, grains as costars, and veggies as the center-stage divas. Animal products should be a side dish or treated as a condiment (if consumed at all), while plant-based foods make up the main course. This very simple and inexpensive change will rock your world, up your life span, and vanquish the scariest C of all—cellulite!

While we're on the topic of thigh cheese, let's dive into a vat of fat for a hot minute. Your body's fat cells are all present by age ten for the most part, but the little buggers are very elastic and can grow in size at any point. A healthy vegetarian or vegan diet consumed in moderate portions helps prevent fat cells from ballooning in size. The recipe for success: Eat lots of high-fiber foods, as many as possible in the raw form, and limit animal products and processed junk. Cellulite is a different beast than overall body fat. As Jennifer Reilly, RD (www.Bitchin Dietitian.com) says, "You can be 'skinny fat' and still have cellulite! Cellulite is formed because of fluid retention and the accumulation of waste products and toxins in the body. The Standard American Diet is very pro-cellulite! Breaking down these foods results in a ton of toxic waste products floating around our systems, and they are visible from the outside in the form of nasty cellulite."

So are you panicked and wondering: "But what about protein? And where will I get my calcium?" Relax and release the fear. The truth is that we can get all the protein and calcium we need from a varied plant-based diet. The healthiest people on the planet are those who eat the fewest animal products. It takes a sexy revolutionary like yourself to buck the system and go your own way. And I promise you, it's worth it. Eat clean and green and toast to life. Cheers!

PREVENTING THE BIG THREE *with Neal D. Barnard, MD*

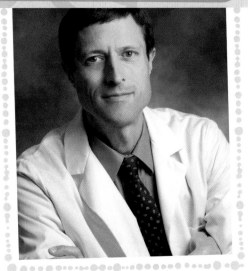

Many people imagine that heart disease, cancer, or diabetes is the natural result of growing older. As the calendar pages turn, we are more and more susceptible to illness, or so many of us think. But let me share some good news. These problems are not caused by the passage of time. No matter how old you are, you can take strong steps to prevent and even reverse these and other serious illnesses. And if these diseases have already struck, there is a lot you can do to turn things around.

A HEALTHY HEART

Heart disease is extremely common. And it often starts very early in life. Many children have the beginnings of heart disease before they pick up their high school diplomas. But if we take a look at what causes it, we'll see how to prevent it—and even how to reverse it. The problem starts with particles of cholesterol flowing along in your bloodstream. These particles irritate the artery wall and cause blister-like bumps—or plaques—to form.

A plaque is fragile and can break open. And when that happens, nearby blood cells react by clumping together in a clot. If the clot plugs the artery, it cuts off the blood supply to the heart itself. A section of the heart muscle dies, which is what we call a "heart attack." Until fairly recently, this process was considered irreversible. A growing plaque was a one-way street leading to the operating room. But Dr. Dean Ornish, a Harvard-trained physician, changed that dismal scenario. He aimed not just to prevent heart disease but to actually reverse it. At

his research center in San Francisco, he asked heart patients to make some powerful lifestyle changes, based on four simple steps:

1. A vegetarian diet. Foods from plants skip the animal fat and cholesterol that lurk in animal products.
2. Regular exercise. That meant a half-hour walk every day, or an hour three times per week.
3. Stress management. This could mean yoga, meditation, or simple breathing or stretching exercises.
4. Avoidance of tobacco.

That was the whole program. There were no drugs, no surgery, no intensive medical treatments of any kind. Easy!

And the results were astounding: Chest pain melted away, and the participants' cholesterol levels plummeted. After a year the research team found something even more dramatic. The participants' arteries had actually opened up, so much so that the difference was clearly visible on angiograms in 82 percent of the people in the study. And the average person had lost more than 20 pounds, which, of course, made them absolutely love the program they had begun.

What are the foods that work this magic? Vegetables, fruits, whole grains, beans, and all the meals that are made from them. So breakfast might be a bowl of old-fashioned oatmeal with cinnamon and raisins. Lunch might be veggie and bean chili with corn bread, and dinner might be pasta marinara with carrots, fresh peas, and onion. Some heart researchers also encourage the use of nuts (say, almonds), soy products, and oats, because each of these is reputed to have special heart-protecting effects.

The foods to avoid are meats, dairy products, eggs, and oily foods. That means throwing out the chicken and fish, too. Yes, fish has some "good" (omega-3) fat. But at least 70 percent of the fat in fish is not "good" fat; it is a mixture of plain old saturated ("bad") fat, along with various other fats that do your heart no good at all. Fish and chicken have too much cholesterol and fat to seriously lower your cholesterol level, they don't help with weight control, and they are not part of the programs that are most powerful for protecting the heart.

PREVENTING CANCER

In the early 1960s researchers made a remarkable observation. People living in certain countries had what seemed to be a measure of protection against cancer. Breast cancer, for example, was common in North America and Europe, but surprisingly rare in Japan. And when cancer did strike Japanese women, they were much more likely to survive than their American or European counterparts.

However, starting in the 1960s, things began to change. Fast foods and meat and cheese business lunches invaded Asia, replacing rice. And cancer rates quickly rose. By the late 1970s Japanese women who had Westernized their diets and ate meat every day had eight times the risk of breast cancer, compared with poorer women who continued traditional rice-based diets. Here's the lesson we can draw: To prevent cancer, it pays to move toward vegetables, fruits, whole grains, and beans.

Part of the value of plant-based diets is that they help us stay slimmer. That is important, because body fat makes estrogens, the female sex hormones that can stimulate cancer growth. Women with less body fat are less likely to develop the common forms of breast cancer, and, if cancer strikes, slimmer women are also more likely to survive. But healthy foods do more than keep us slim. Two large studies put diet changes to the test. Their goal was not to see if cancer could be prevented, but to see what foods could do to help women who had already had breast cancer. The Women's Intervention Nutrition Study (WINS), including nearly 2,500 post-menopausal women who had previously been treated for cancer, showed that cutting down on fatty foods did indeed reduce the odds that their cancer would come back. The Women's Healthy Eating and Living (WHEL) study, which included more than 3,000 women, showed that a combination of a diet very rich in vegetables and fruits, along with regular exercise, could cut the risk of a recurrence in half.

The lesson we draw from these studies is that avoiding fatty foods and bringing in the vegetables and fruits, along with physical activity, can make a huge difference. If these healthy changes can help women who have already had cancer, they are likely to be even more powerful before cancer strikes.

DIABETES

Diabetes is getting to be so common, we would call it a fad if it weren't so dangerous. In simple terms, diabetes means there is too much sugar in the blood. The sugar we are thinking of here is glucose, which is supposed to provide energy for your body. It powers your brain, your muscles, and other organs. But in diabetes, glucose is having trouble getting into the cells where it belongs. Instead it builds up in the bloodstream, where it can damage the delicate blood vessels of your eyes, kidneys, heart, and legs. Needless to say, you don't want that to happen.

Why is glucose having trouble getting into the cells? Why is it building up in the bloodstream? Let me draw an analogy: To get through the front door of your house, you use a key. What if you were to arrive home one day to find that your key does not turn in your lock? You look carefully at the key, and it is clear that there is nothing wrong with it. But looking into the lock, you discover that, while you were away, someone stuck gum in it. You could spend the rest of your life crawling in and out of the window. But it would make more sense to clean out the lock.

When glucose enters your cells, it uses a "key," too. Glucose's key is insulin, a hormone that opens tiny channels in the cell's outer membrane, allowing glucose to pass through. But in Type 2 diabetes, the common form of diabetes that affects so many people nowadays, the insulin key isn't working properly. Researchers have looked into why insulin is not able to open up the cell, and what they have found has dramatically changed our view of diabetes.

It turns out that your cells can get gummed up, too. Just as gum in a lock interferes with a key, fat particles from the foods you eat can enter the cells and interfere with insulin's ability to open the cell membrane to glucose. The answer to diabetes is to clean out your cells. When you avoid fatty foods, it is like cleaning gum out of a lock. Fat leaves your cells, and insulin starts to work better.

In our research, we have found that simple dietary changes can do the trick, dramatically improving diabetes. In some cases people improve so much that no one would know they had ever had the condition.

There are three keys to preventing diabetes (or reversing it if you have it now):

1. Avoid all animal products.
2. Keep vegetable oils to a minimum.
3. Avoid sugar and refined flour products.

These simple steps can help your cells to clean themselves out, reversing the process that leads to diabetes. We do not limit how many calories or carbohydrate grams you choose, so you'll never go hungry. And the foods you eat are all good for you. As you'll notice, they are similar to the ones that reversed heart disease and caused dramatic weight loss in Dr. Ornish's study.

So although heart problems, cancer, and diabetes are serious problems, they have nothing to do with how old we are. They relate to how long and how badly we have been abusing our bodies. If we give ourselves healthful foods, exercise, and the healthful environment we need, we can prevent these problems to a great extent. And if you already have encountered one of these health challenges, foods can help you heal.

Neal D. Barnard, MD, best-selling author of *Food for Life, Dr. Neal Barnard's Program for Reversing Diabetes,* and other titles, is the founder of Physicians Committee for Responsible Medicine (PCRM), a group that promotes preventive medicine and addresses controversies in modern medicine.

OMNIVORE OR HERBIVORE?

"But wait!" you say. "We've been eating body parts for ages, what's the problem?" True. While our ancestors have been eating meat since they came down from the trees, they consumed it infrequently and in smaller portions. Also, the meat was very different. It was wild and fresh, not from disease-ridden factory farms that dose already sick animals with drugs and chemicals. Though we were hunter-gatherers, we gathered a heck of a lot more than we hunted. Woolly mammoth was a luxury saved for special occasions, like bar mitzvahs and weddings.

Many nutrition experts believe that humans are ill equipped to fully digest and absorb meat. Though we're practicing omnivores, we appear to be more like herbivores physiologically. The true question: What's optimal? The true answer: Plants.

Consider a carnivore, the lovely lioness. She has claws, fangs, and an abundance of hydrochloric acid to do the tough job of digesting flesh. I don't know about you, but I'm not gonna chip my manicure attacking and gutting Bessie the cow. Humans have molars and masticating jaws, perfect for grinding and chewing high-fiber goodies. Our stomachs contain hydrochloric acid in smaller amounts better designed to digest plant proteins.

In addition, the lioness dines on fresh kill, preferably organs high in minerals. Because she doesn't haul around a camping stove, Madame Lioness eats her food raw and therefore receives all the enzymatic benefits. Her short digestive tract ensures that zebra goes in, zebra comes out. Now think of the length of our intestines, about 26 twisting, curving feet. Pig goes in; pig stays in for days and weeks at a time. Pig makes us bloated and bitchy. Our personal thermostat hovers around 98.6. What happens to pig at that temperature? Stink city! If our digestive fires aren't strong, the former Being rots and corrupts our internal environment. Bad bacteria go wild; it's like their version of a coke whore bender.

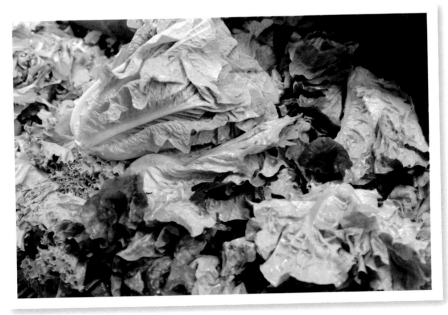

PROTEIN: THE MYTH AND THE MAGIC

The belief that we need enormous amounts of protein to be healthy and strong is one of the most pervasive myths in America. In fact, overdosing on protein is one of the key reasons why we've become so unhealthy. Studies show that as protein consumption goes up, so do the rates of chronic disease. In truth, protein deficiency is virtually nonexistent in industrialized countries. Walk around any Uncle Sam strip mall and you'll see that our problem is quite different: a full-blown obesity epidemic. Obesity is just one of many casualties of a country suffocating under the burden of diseases of affluence. What do I mean by diseases of affluence? This term commonly describes the maladies that are killing our friends, families, neighbors, and coworkers. Historically, the rich could afford meat, cream, saturated fat, rich sweets, and spirits. Yet, the more they consumed the more health problems they experienced. Now thanks to the availability of fast cheap food (which you'll learn about it in a hot second), we can all afford to break down and fall apart. Underdeveloped nations have their problems, too. But they tend to concentrate around sanitation, safe drinking water, and basic medicines. Cultures that rely on traditional plant-based diets have far fewer cases of the big diseases that we all fear.

As gardens are being replaced by test tubes, the American public has become one big science experiment. The Standard American Diet is tap dancing on the last nerve of our health. And in the age of rapid globalization, SAD has spread like an aggressive cancer. As a result, the major health issues that are soaring in our country are now plaguing the entire planet. Thank you, Uncle Sam, for the globalization of illness. Bravo!

We're digging our graves with our forks and steak knives. And check this out: Many average to overweight people are actually malnourished! Whoa, how is that possible? Excess animal protein and fat clog your cells, bloodstream, and colon. As a result, you absorb less nutrition from your food. In addition, poor-quality grub leaves us still feeling hungry. So what do we do? Eat more, get less, and gain weight.

Is protein important? Absolutely, but in large quantities it's deadly. In his book *Eat Right America,* Joel Fuhrman, a renowned MD and nutrition expert, likens our extreme emphasis on protein to dietary suicide. He suggests that unless you're anorexic, you don't have to worry about consuming enough protein. The trick is to upgrade the proteins we consume and to make safer choices on a regular basis.

HOW MUCH PROTEIN DO YOU REALLY NEED?

The USDA's recommended daily allowance is about 0.36 gram of protein for every pound of body weight. So let's say you're that mythical 130-pound woman nutritionists always use as an example. In that case, you need about 47 grams of protein (130 x 0.36) every day. But many experts believe this recommendation is too high. Dr. Furhman suggests that we only need about 20 to 35 grams of protein per day.

How does that compare with reality? The average American adult consumes between 100 and 120 grams of protein every day. Not only is that nearly five times what we need, it comes mostly from high-fat animal products. But just for the sake of argument, let's go with the government's standards. What do 47 grams of protein look like? It doesn't

B ALL THAT YOU CAN B

Vitamin B_{12} is needed for cell division and blood formation. Neither plants nor animals make it, but bacteria do. Animals get it when they munch on foods contaminated with bacteria that generate B_{12}, and in turn the animal becomes a source of the vitamin. Plant foods don't naturally contain enough B_{12} except perhaps when they are contaminated by microorganisms—but since we wash our veggies when we get home (which is a good thing), the microorganisms are washed away.

Crazy Sexy Diet followers should take supplements to get vitamin B_{12} in their diet. Although the need for vitamin B_{12} is quite small, a deficiency is a serious problem that can result in anemia and irreversible nerve damage. Certain fermented foods contain B_{12}, and so does fortified nutritional yeast, but you might not be able to get the amount you need. My advice: Stick with a supplement. Read chapter 9 for more information.

take much: $1/4$ cup almonds contains 7.4 grams, $1/2$ cup quinoa contains 3 grams, $1/2$ cup tempeh contains 15.8 grams, 1 cup lentils contains 17.9 grams, 1 cup broccoli contains 2.6 grams.

So clearly, if you're eating a well-balanced vegetarian diet—meaning you're consuming a wide variety of high-quality foods, like vegetables, greens, sprouts, legumes, tempeh, beans, nuts, grains, and so on—then you will certainly meet your protein needs. Pregnant or breast-feeding women need more protein, as do athletes. But even these needs can easily be met just by eating more of the good stuff. Talk with a holistic-minded doctor or naturopath to make sure you're getting what you need.

> **If you're eating a well-balanced vegetarian diet—meaning you're consuming a wide variety of high-quality foods, like vegetables, greens, sprouts, legumes, tempeh, beans, nuts, grains, and so on—then you will certainly meet your protein needs.**

COMPLETE PROTEINS

Proteins are long strings of amino acids. There are twenty different amino acids you need for good health, but our bodies can only make eleven of them. The remaining nine are referred to as essential amino acids. Because we can't make them, it is essential for us to get them from our diet. Foods that contain all nine essential aminos are known as complete proteins. However, labeling foods as having either "complete" or "incomplete" proteins plays into the idea that some proteins are better for you than others.

While animal flesh is a complete protein, it's also "complete" with saturated fat, cholesterol, hormones, antibiotics, and other unsavory party poopers like *E. coli*. Human flesh is actually the most complete source of protein for us because the amino acids are already in the ideal proportions, but that doesn't mean I should eat the FedEx guy. Unlike their vegetarian counterparts, animal proteins are high in saturated fat, are very acidic, and lack phytonutrients, water, antioxidants, enzymes, and fiber.

Newsflash: Many plants have complete proteins, too! Can you say quinoa, soy products, buckwheat, and hemp seeds? Other plant proteins are only slightly incomplete, so as long as you're eating a variety of them you've got a complete protein powerhouse. You don't even have to eat them all at the same meal or even on the same day. The great Goddess would have shot you out of your mom's Vjay with a calculator and food chart if nature intended you to worry about grams of protein and combining grains and legumes at every meal.

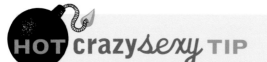

HOT crazysexy TIP

Worried that you won't get enough iron on the CSD? Don't be. You'll get plenty with a varied plant-based diet. Studies show that vegans consume as much iron as omnivores, and sometimes more. In fact, foods with vitamin C boost iron absorption big time. You'll be getting lots of vitamin C with all the raw foods and green juices on the Crazy Sexy Diet. Since you're avoiding coffee and tea (especially with meals), you'll also avoid their tannins, which inhibit iron absorption. Tofu, chickpeas, pinto beans, soybeans, spinach, lentils, pumpkin seeds, Swiss chard, and dried apricots are a few iron-rich plant foods.

PLANT FOODS HIGH IN PROTEIN

Food	Amount	Protein in grams
Almonds	¼ cup	7.4
Barley, pearled	½ cup	3.6
Black beans	1 cup	15
Black-eyed peas	1 cup	13
Broccoli	1 cup, ckd	5
Brown rice	1 cup, ckd	9
Cashews	¼ cup	5
Chickpeas	1 cup	15
Corn	1 cup	5
Cranberry beans	1 cup	17
Flaxseeds	2 T	4
Hemp seeds	3 T	15
Kale	1 cup, ckd	2
Kidney beans	1 cup	15
Lentils	1 cup	18
Lima beans	1 cup	15
Millet	1 cup	8
Natto	½ cup	15
Navy beans	1 cup	16
Oatmeal	1 cup, ckd	6
Peas	1 cup	9
Peanut butter	2 T	7
Peanuts	1 ounce	7
Pinto beans	1 cup	14
Potato, baked	1 medium	4
Quinoa	1 cup, ckd	6
Spinach	1 cup, ckd	5
Sunflower seeds	1 ounce	6
Sweet potato, baked	1 medium	2
Tempeh	1 cup	30
Tofu, firm	4 ounces	10
Walnuts	1 ounce	4

For more information, I recommend brendadavisrd.com.

GOT PROPAGANDA?

Okay, it's time for a rant. Now, don't get me wrong. If you're going for 60/40 and you'll just snap and dump the CSD altogether if you can't add a bit of raw goat cheese (from a safe, quality source) to your salad, then by all means fit it in. I'd rather you ate a small portion of better-quality dairy and stayed on track. However, I've got a beef with the dairy industry, and maybe after you read this section you'll have one too. Good-bye creamer, hello hemp milk!

The meat and dairy industries spend a fortune to keep their products synonymous with good health. They do it directly to consumers through sophisticated ad campaigns using lots of glam celebs, but they also do it indirectly by influencing government. Industry executives become government regulators then become industry executives again, like one big revolving door swirling with crazy money. As a result, the official regulations and guidelines that are so influential to public health are often compromised. While confusion and misinformation benefit stockholders, they don't always protect our best interests or our children's.

Take, for example, federal school lunch programs. They have two conflicting aims: better health for kids and boosting agriculture industries. Unfortunately, under the current system, the lion's share of spending goes to the unhealthy meat, dairy, and egg products. So is it any surprise that these government meals routinely fail their own government nutritional standards? In an attempt to buck this BS, in 2009 Baltimore city schools decided to participate in the popular "Meatless Monday" campaign—the first in the country to do so. What's the problem with a little veggie chili? Well, the mad cowboys went on a cable news butchering spree.

The American Meat Institute had the balls to imply that their products were the only real source of protein and that one meatless meal per week was putting our kids in harm's way. Last time I checked, childhood obesity and diabetes are more dangerous than a bowl of veggie chili.

Sophisticated marketing campaigns and manipulative language have an enormous impact on the foods we buy. "Got milk?" or how about "Milk: It does the body good." You've probably seen those ads a gazillion times. Here's some poetry for ya: "Milk is milk." Huh? Yeah, those three little words are supposed to convince us that there is no difference between "natural" milk and milk from cows injected with Monsanto's genetically engineered growth hormones.

What if I told you that you've been eating lies and propaganda? Would you get mad? I certainly would. I certainly am. When I was a kid, schoolteachers drilled the importance of tits and ass into my head. The food pyramid ruled. Well, guess who supplied our classrooms with teaching materials? The National Dairy Council.

Today the National Dairy Council invests millions of dollars every year in the "Got Milk" campaign. The message: If you drink from the almighty animal mammary, you too can be rich, skinny, and successful, just like your favorite celebrity. It's dangerous when uninformed celebrities don the mustache and lead the masses down an unhealthy road. Where are the actors, athletes, and rock stars willing to stand up for broccoli? Can you imagine what would happen if Leo and Clooney wore EAT KALE, NOT COW tees on the red carpet? How about a GOT NUT MILK? hoodie? I'd love to see Gwen Stefani or Fergie stroll to her workout in one of those.

WEAN!

A cow drinks cow's milk when it's a baby. A bunny drinks bunny's milk when it's a baby. Beyond a certain age, even they know that it's freaky to suckle. And do you ever see them switch and swap? The only time milk is essential for good health is when we are babies, being breast-fed by human mothers. Human breast milk is nature's perfect formula for human babies. It's rich in good fats like DHA for brain development, but it's relatively low in protein. Cow's milk contains more than three times as much protein as breast milk. That's because baby cows need a lot more protein. They grow to between 1,500 and 2,000 pounds. Is that your desired weight? If so, hello reality TV!

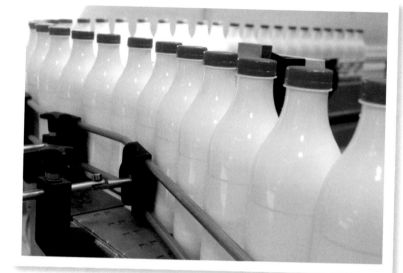

Leonid Shcheglov

While the protein in human milk is designed for human bodies, much of the protein in cow's milk is difficult for humans to digest. Dr. T. Colin Campbell, professor emeritus of nutritional biochemistry at Cornell University, is a pioneering researcher in the investigation of the diet–cancer link. Put his book *The China Study* on your must-read list today! It clears up the fallacies of our modern diet and provides a thought-provoking look at what really causes cancer. Here's the CliffsNotes version: One of the biggest contenders is a diet containing more than 10 percent protein (that's about 50 grams of protein if you're consuming 2,000 calories per day). Americans eat way more than that (an average of 17 percent total protein, of which 12 to 13 percent is animal-based!). Dr. Campbell found that the protein that consistently creates and promotes cancer is casein, which makes up 87 percent of the protein in cow's milk.

His research verifies that the types of protein that don't promote cancer, even at high levels of intake, are the safe proteins from plants. Dr. Campbell writes, "In fact, dietary protein proved to be so powerful in its effect that they could turn on and turn off cancer growth simply by changing the level consumed." Did you read that correctly? Turn off cancer cells, go veg! Dr. Campbell estimates that "80 to 90 percent of all cancers, cardiovascular diseases, and other degenerative illness can be prevented, at least until very old age, simply by adopting a plant-based diet."

Forget spooky, life-threatening diseases, let's talk about simpler pickles. Ever pass a kidney stone? If you have, then you know that it's incredibly painful—sorta feels like you're shitting an elephant through your pee hole! How about Crohn's disease, a veritable pain and inflammation blow-out sale? Both of these not-so-happy afflictions have been linked to dairy consumption. Allergies, eczema, asthma, arthritis, inflammation, and zits can all be linked to dairy. What about skim milk or nonfat milk? They're just as bad. For me, cheese was the hardest thing to give up, but once I did, my weird rashes and forehead bumps disappeared. I also started to breathe easier—a pretty important change for a gal with cancer in her lungs. Perhaps this is too much information, but my poo changed, too. It came out regularly and stopped being coated in mucus. (More on that in chapter 5, lucky you!)

How about tummy pain and intestinal gas and bloating? Well, there may be a good reason for your belly's aching. According to the American Academy of Family Physicians, around 75 percent of the world's adults can't digest milk (they're lactose-intolerant). Among some populations, such as Native Americans and Asians, the figure is close to 100 percent. Beyond childhood, most people stop producing the enzyme lactase, which is needed to digest lactose (the sugar in milk). Yeah, your body thinks you should wean, too. I've never met someone who didn't feel better once they removed dairy from their diet. Sorry folks, but all good things come to an end.

STRONG BONES with Lilli B. Link, MD

If you are wondering if being a vegan is okay for your bones, don't worry—a small but credible study suggests that it is. In this study the people following the raw vegan diet were much thinner and had lower bone density (which goes along with being thinner). The reassuring part of the study was that the blood markers of bone turnover (how much bone was formed and broken down) showed no difference between those who followed the raw vegan diet and those who followed a typical American diet that contained almost twice the amount of calcium as the raw vegan diet. In other words, the people on the vegan diet weren't losing bone mass any faster than those eating animal food.

According to the National Academy of Sciences (NAS), the recommended intake of calcium for adults is 1,000 to 1,200 milligrams a day, depending on your age and gender. It's hard to consume that much calcium if you don't eat any dairy products, but contrary to popular belief, you don't need milk for strong bones and good health—and you may not need as much dietary calcium as you think, despite what the NAS and the USDA say.

In a recent study that compared calcium consumption in different countries, the countries with the lowest calcium intake (about 500 to 1,000 mg/day), such as Yugoslavia and Singapore, had lower rates of hip fractures (the dreaded outcome of low bone density) than the countries with the highest calcium intake (over 1,000 mg/day), such as the United States and New Zealand. Another study published in 2000 showed that countries with the highest consumption of animal protein intake had the most hip fractures, whereas the countries with the highest vegetable protein intake had the fewest hip fractures. So much for needing calcium from animal foods to keep your bones strong!

Since people from other countries who eat much less calcium than we do have fewer fractures, maybe it's not all about how much calcium we eat. What's more important is how much we keep from what we eat. Two other nutrients particularly affect how much calcium

LEAN ON ME:
WEIGHT-BEARING EXERCISE

Your bones don't thrive on calcium alone. One of the best ways to avoid bone loss and build bone density is to do some heavy lifting. Just twelve to twenty minutes of strength-training, weight-bearing, or resistance exercise three days a week, say researchers at the Bone & Joint Injury Prevention & Rehabilitation Center at the University of Michigan, can increase bone density.

Weight-bearing exercise stimulates bone formation and calcium retention. Walking, weight lifting, jogging, hiking, yoga, aerobics, dancing, and working out on the treadmill, elliptical trainer, or stair-stepper are just a few of the fun games you can give your bones. Pick your favorite(s) and commit consistently. If you're trying something new, find a pro to guide you so you know the proper form. PS: Swimming and biking don't count. The water and wheels shield you from one very important thing: gravity.

we hold on to: protein and sodium. The more protein and sodium we eat, the more calcium we urinate out.

It follows, then, that if we eat less protein and sodium (we consume high levels of both in the course of a day, especially because salt is often hidden in processed foods), we probably don't need to eat as much calcium. Good plant sources of calcium are dark green vegetables such as broccoli, collard greens, and kale, along with nuts and seeds. A diet rich in these foods and low in animal protein and salt should provide enough calcium to keep your bones strong.

The other side of the equation is the absorption of calcium. It's better absorbed when eaten along with vitamin C. That means that the vitamin-C-loaded lemon juice on your green leafy vegetable is helping you absorb the vegetable's calcium (and the vegetable itself has plenty of vitamin C as well).

If you need some added incentive to cut dairy foods from your diet, read on. As a result of the milking process, cows often have mastitis (an infection of the udder), making their milk full of white blood cells, aka pus. This means milk-based foods, such as butter, yogurt, cottage cheese, all kinds of hard cheeses, ice cream, and so on, are often also full of pus.

In addition to the foods you know are made from milk, there are some ingredients you might not know are dairy-based: whey (used in protein powder mixes), casein (used in protein powders and some rice

PLANT FOODS HIGH IN CALCIUM

Food	Amount	Calcium in mg
Almonds, dry-roasted	1 ounce	80
Arugula	½ cup	16
Black beans	1 cup	60
Broccoli, cooked	1 cup	42
Cabbage, cooked	½ cup	25
Chickpeas	1 cup	80
Collard greens, cooked	½ cup	113
Cranberry beans	1 cup	89
Flaxseeds	1 ounce	48
Kale, cooked	½ cup	90
Kidney beans	1 cup	50
Lentils	1 cup	38
Natto	½ cup	190
Navy beans	1 cup	128
Okra	½ cup	50
Peanuts	1 ounce	15
Pinto beans	1 cup	82
Potato, baked	1 medium	20
Quinoa	1 cup	102
Spinach, cooked	½ cup, raw	30*
Sunflower seeds	1 ounce	34
Sweet potato, baked	1 medium	32
Swiss chard, cooked	½ cup	30*
Tahini	1 ounce	128
Tempeh	1 cup	184
Tofu	½ cup	130
Turnip greens, cooked	½ cup	99

* Spinach, chard, beet greens, and rhubarb are not the best sources for calcium, because they contain high amounts of oxalates that bind minerals and make calcium unavailable

For more information, I recommend brendadavisrd.com.

and soy cheeses), kefir (a fermented milk drink sort of like yogurt), ghee (often used in Indian food), lactalbumin, and lactose. An even longer list of manufactured food additives come from dairy, but once you get into names that are so unfamiliar (and hard to pronounce!), you probably shouldn't be eating that product.

If you buy the whole food, you don't have to worry about what's been added to it. Some people argue that raw dairy is much healthier than milk that has been pasteurized and homogenized. Not really—lactose is lactose and pus is pus. And although it is uncommon, people can also get sick from the bacteria in raw milk.

It's been ten years since I've had dairy of any kind, and at this point I no longer even miss the cheese that sits on top of my former favorite food: pizza. But if you think you need some milk or cheese substitutes, at least during the transition period of your diet change, there are plenty of good vegan (soy-, rice-, or tapioca-based) and raw (nut- or seed-based) options to satisfy your palate.

Lilli B. Link, MD, MS, is a board-certified internist currently practicing as a nutritional counselor in New York City. She specializes in raw foods and integrative nutrition. Visit her at www.llinkmd.com.

HORMONES

I don't know about you, but I'm a child of the '70s. Back in my groovy day, girls requested training bras for their newly sprouted titties at around thirteen or fourteen years of age. I'll never forget my "period party" celebration dinner at the Ming Hoy Chinese restaurant (just me and my parents, ugh). Today kids as young as eight are developing into Pam Anderson–stacked rugby players. Not only is it unnatural, it's dangerous. Let's look at some possible reasons.

Steroids are widely—and legally—used in the beef, pork, and poultry industries, because they make the animals grow bigger faster. How about hormones? You betcha! In order to make milk all year round, Bessie the cow gets dosed with hormones so she'll stay constantly knocked up and lactating—a living milk machine. (Damn, I would be such an uncomfortable wench!)

She's also injected with recombinant bovine growth hormone (rBGH) to double her milk production. This synthetic cocktail increases another hormone, IGF-1, which, as you learned in chapter 3, is linked to the big C. Because she's a baby factory, a cow makes way more estrogen than nature intended—and it comes out in her milk. In the United States dairy products account for 60 to 80 percent of estrogens consumed!

In 2008 Harvard researchers studied the effect of giving US commercial milk to third-graders in Mongolia. After drinking it for a month, their growth hormone levels shot up 40 percent. The children actually grew about 1 centimeter during the month, a significant statistical change, according to the researchers. Those bright Harvard minds are currently studying whether growth spurts from milk will affect sexual maturity and puberty age. What do you think?

According to researchers at the US Centers for Disease Control and Prevention, in Westernized societies, girls who get their periods before the age of twelve and who have the most menstrual cycles over a lifetime have a higher risk of dying from ovarian cancer than women with fewer period cycles. The same seems to be true of breast cancer. Earlier puberty means more menstrual cycles—and hormone-laced milk, meat, and poultry are associated with bringing on the acne years at a younger age. Childhood obesity also triggers puberty sooner—and kids who consume dairy products and meat tend to be overweight. You can see the way industrial protein production can lead to a disease spiral that starts in childhood.

When I follow the trail, it sure seems like conventional dairy products are more harmful than helpful. My fear is that by the time science has it figured out, we'll have lost too many of our mothers, sisters, and wives. If you're only willing to give up one thing, put dairy at the top of the list. Ya think the boys are off the hook? Not so fast, Frankie. Excess estrogen not only makes boys mature later and have man-boobs, but it can also delay emotional development . . . let the dating disasters begin! And if they make it into the backseat, not to worry: Estrogen is being examined as a possible culprit in declining sperm counts.

Okay, one more hormone rant and I swear I'm done. Got rage? Speaking from experience, I know what it's like when stress hormones like adrenaline and cortisol explode through my body. I have plenty of work to do controlling my fear and white-hot temper tantrums. I don't need any additional stress, thank you very much! When cows are being forced into kill chutes at the slaughterhouse, you better believe they know what's about to happen. The absolute panic forces their bodies to release tons of fight-or-flight hormones, which flood their tissues. When you eat their meat, you're getting those hormones as well. Not good. I call it chemical karma.

C IS FOR CARCINOGENIC

Let's move on to something far more uplifting: carcinogens! Cooked meat increases the risk of developing . . . what else? You guessed it, cancer! Gold star. Even the National Cancer Institute and the American Institute for Cancer Research (AICR) verify that little gem. It's because cooking meat, especially at high temperatures like on the barbecue grill, under the broiler, or in the deep fryer, creates nasty substances called heterocyclic amines (HCAs). The more well done the meat, the more HCAs it has, and the more carcinogenic it becomes. HCAs are known to cause stomach cancer and also breast, colon, and pancreatic cancer.

THE SKINNY ON ATKINS *with Alejandro Junger, MD*

It is curious that nutrition, the most basic of human needs, is the one we often know the least about, doctors included. Until recently, most medical schools did not even offer, let alone require, the study of diets and nutrition. The lack of unified thinking about nutrition is the perfect climate for toxic ideas and urban legends to spread like weeds, and worse—to be put into practice by whole populations. The perfect example of such a phenomenon is the Atkins diet.

In 1972 Dr. Robert Atkins published his book *Dr. Atkins' Diet Revolution,* the most popular of a subsequent wave of high-protein, low-carb diet titles. The high-protein, low-carb craze that ruled the '80s and '90s still lingers, despite ample, unequivocal scientific proof that it leads to high acidity and

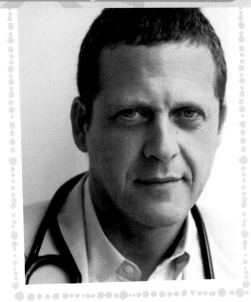

thus is a contributing factor to heart disease, cancer, and the rest of the chronic diseases.

Understanding the context in which the Atkins diet took over America, and was imported by every other country in the world, may help us avoid repeating such costly mistakes in the future. Here are some of the reasons why Atkins exploded and what they reveal about our culture:

- **HISTORICAL CONTEXT.** In the 1970s America had just been deceived by the first mass diet movement, the low-fat madness. Eliminating fat from our lives promised to be the solution to excess weight, but instead, it resulted in the fattest country in the world. The food industry saturated the market with low-fat and no-fat foods. The calories and flavor missing as a result of fat elimination were replaced with calories from carbohydrates. The result was weight gain, not weight loss. The war on fat was being lost. America needed new generals, but most importantly, it needed a new enemy. Almost overnight we went from no fat to no carbs, the new enemy.

- **THE MD FACTOR.** America loves doctors. We watch them on TV shows obsessively. Dr. Atkins had the most important ingredient when it comes to gaining popular trust, the letters MD after his name. Gullibility is a silent American epidemic.

- **EFFECTIVENESS.** Results rule, and Atkins delivers its promise: weight loss from fat burning. This leads to a leaner body. America's obsession with being skinny overrides its concerns for being healthy. This of course was strategically marketed by the Atkins brand. Dr. Atkins knew that depriving the body of carbohydrates forces the metabolism to activate its survival mechanisms. Our cells work best when they burn glucose from carbohydrates to generate energy.

  If carbs go missing, the body uses stored fat as the next best fuel. When fatty acids are broken down by the liver and kidneys to be used for fuel, ketone bodies are one of the by-products. The presence of ketone bodies results in a condition known as ketosis. A low level of ketosis, created by fasting briefly, by going on a very low-calorie diet, or even in the morning after not eating overnight, is common. But when large amounts of ketones rapidly accumulate in the blood, as can happen to people with Type 1 diabetes who don't get their insulin, the condition is called keto-acidosis—a medical emergency. The body is designed to use ketones as a temporary solution to a shortage of glucose. Being constantly in ketosis, however, can make your blood acidic, because the molecular composition of ketones resembles alcohol.

There's nothing revolutionary about using the ketosis metabolic pathway to burn fat. Body-builders were using it decades before Atkins wrote about it as a way to lose weight. The overall systemic acidity that inevitably results from a high-protein, low-carb diet helps you lose weight but has long-term negative consequences, including inflammation, chronic digestive problems, heart disease, and cancer.

If your goal is rapid weight loss, Atkins works well. It's a short-term approach, however. If your goal is to achieve wellness and longevity, you need a long-term approach that avoids systemic acidity. A diet with no animal products and plenty of fresh vegetables and whole grains avoids acidity and is satisfying while also being high in nutrients and lower in calories. You can lose weight safely while improving, not damaging, your health.

Alejandro Junger, MD, is the best-selling author of *Clean: The Revolutionary Program to Restore the Body's Natural Ability to Heal Itself.*

P IS FOR PROCESSED

Processed meats are the worst offenders against our bods. You can and should really do without them. The fare typically served at ballparks, Mafia meetings, and in your cozy breakfast nook I call "L&A meats" because they're made of lips and assholes—all the leftover stuff too gross for other uses. I'm talking about bologna, pastrami, and salami, as well as hot dogs and sausages, to which carcinogenic nitrates and other chemicals have been added.

This isn't breaking news to most people. I certainly didn't think it was a hot topic until I mentioned this information during a speech I gave at a well-respected children's hospital. After my speech, I was asked to sit on a panel. A lovely young girl raised her hand. She had brain cancer and was concerned about recent findings on the connection between cell phones and tumors. The doctor sitting to my left answered her question very snootily, "Please, there's no connection. Use your cell phone . . . and eat your hot dogs, too, for that matter." I received the doctor's message loud and clear, as well as her dirty look (which I wanted to smack off her face, but my mother raised a lady!). One week later I received a copy of *Good Medicine,* the quarterly magazine of the Physicians Committee for Responsible Medicine (PCRM). Check out the title of the lead article in the issue: "Expelled! Processed Meats Cause Cancer. So Why Do Schools Feed Them to Children?" I only wish I was armed with that issue at the podium that day.

That a doctor in a major metropolitan hospital could be so out of touch was astounding. The evidence is overwhelming, and even heavy hitters like the American Cancer Institute and the World Cancer Research Fund agree that no amount of processed meat is healthy; it therefore should be avoided completely. In fact, the risk of colorectal cancer increases by 21 percent for every 50 grams of processed meat consumed daily. Keep in mind that 50 grams is about one hot dog. Other studies have also linked processed meats to cancer of the esophagus, lung, stomach, and prostate. Yet these products are still widely consumed. According to the National Hot Dog & Sausage Council, more than 740 million hot dog packages were sold in 2007. A truckload of which is chowed down each year at the Coney Island hot-dog-eating contest. Boy, is that a gold-star event—the Super Bowl of Gratuitous Gluttony. "Look, world, I ate sixty-eight hot dogs in ten minutes! And as a reward, I get this handsome trophy and a colostomy bag. Gee whiz, dreams really do come true."

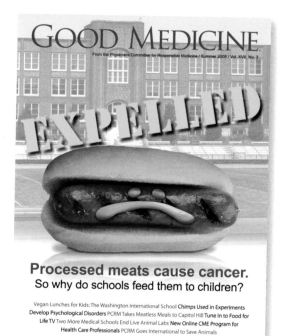

Processed meats cause cancer.
So why do schools feed them to children?

Vegan Lunches for Kids: The Washington International School **Chimps Used in Experiments Develop Psychological Disorders** PCRM Takes Meatless Meals to Capitol Hill **Tune In to Food for Life TV** Two More Medical Schools End Live Animal Labs **New Online CME Program for Health Care Professionals** PCRM Goes International to Save Animals

THE REAL COST OF MEAT

Wow—99-cent burgers at the drive-through! A bucket of chicken for pocket change! What a deal! Or is it? From the fast-food window to the supermarket deli counter, the true price of meat in America is actually much higher than what we pay at the register. That's because behind every pound of flesh sold there is a cascade of hidden costs to our health, economy, and environment.

It takes enormous amounts of resources to raise beef cattle in our factory farm system. To fatten them rapidly, the critters are fed huge amounts of growth hormones and cheap corn. But there's one problem: Nature designed them to eat grass. Understandably, their modified diet causes all sorts of health problems, which require antibiotics and other drugs. Their health suffers further from often filthy and overcrowded living conditions, meaning more and more antibiotics. A cow can be so unhealthy by slaughter time, it probably would have died of disease soon after anyway.

Government policies play a big role in keeping meat cheap. Subsidies—your tax dollars—pay farmers to grown way more feed corn than is needed, which results in mountains of rotting food and unrealistically low prices. Some even say that the sharp rise in meat consumption we've seen over the past few decades was actually caused by all that extra corn looking for a customer!

Subsidies are also filtered through land-use policy. Ranchers who lease public land reap the profits, but we taxpayers pick up the tab for environmental damage. And last but not least, governments love to give tax breaks to anyone promising to bring jobs to town. But the jobs aren't so great. According to MarketWatch, slaughterhouse workers are among the top ten most underpaid in the US.

Unfortunately, they also suffer some of the highest injury rates.

Ever wonder why there are so many recalls of meat because of *E. coli* or salmonella contamination? The industrial meat system is ground zero for foodborne illnesses. Yum, bacteria on a bun! According to the Centers for Disease Control and Prevention, 76 million Americans are sickened from foodborne illnesses each year. Animal feces are a primary cause, either in meats directly or by contact with the crops grown near the animals. That was the case with the big spinach outbreak a few years ago. The investigation found the likely cause was wild boars that rooted in the cattle lots, then wandered down-valley to poop on the spinach. Of course, the cattle folks did everything they could to blame the spinach.

Massive slaughterhouses, which can kill thousands of Beings per day, are a germ invasion. Bessie is disemboweled and often, in the assembly-line rush, her guts get punctured and fecal matter seeps onto her flesh. This is particularly dangerous with hamburger because when the meat is ground, the pathogens get mixed and spread. Besides that, there's no such thing as one cow on your plate. Lord only knows how many creatures from how many factories went into that happy meal—it's kinda like an *E. coli* smoothie. It takes only a tiny number of bacteria to cause serious illness. And guess who gets it the worst? Old people and kids.

It's no secret that America is in the midst of a health care crisis, as rising costs threaten to bankrupt our entire economy. And as you've already learned, we also have an obesity epidemic. These distinct problems are actually two sides of the same coin, and you can't fix one without addressing the other. The CDC estimates that the health care price tag of obesity in 2008 was $147 billion—more than doubling in less than a decade. Meat is public enemy number one in heart disease, strokes, and many cancers. And cornfed meat is much higher in saturated fat than meat from cows that graze on grass, their natural food.

The health effects of chemicals and toxins are harder to estimate, but the cost in dollars and lives is certainly enormous. The industrial food system dumps millions of tons of pollutants into our environment every year. Feedlots and farms are responsible for much of it: hormones, medicines, infected fecal waste, fertilizers, and pesticides all end up in our soil and waterways. Ever hear of a dead zone? It's an area of water that is effectively dead of marine life. Nada, kaput. It's caused when fertilizers flow downriver from farms and choke out oxygen. There's a dead zone in the Gulf of Mexico the size of New Jersey and at least 400 others around the world.

In 2006 the United Nations released a report called "Livestock's Long Shadow." It revealed that animal agriculture is responsible for more greenhouse gas emissions each year than all the planes, trains, boats, cars, and trucks on earth. Meat production was believed to account for some 18 percent of the world's total emissions. But scientists have since been revising that estimate upward. In 2009 the World Bank put out a new report that pegged it at 51 percent—more than all other sources combined!

Methane gas from animal poo and farts is a big problem. Methane is twenty-one times more harmful to the atmosphere than CO_2. Also contributing to global warming is the bulldozing and burning of rain forest to make way for animal agriculture. In Brazil and elsewhere, lush forests are giving way to barren landscapes for either grazing cattle or growing crops to feed the cattle. Trees act as "carbon sinks" because they inhale and store carbon dioxide.

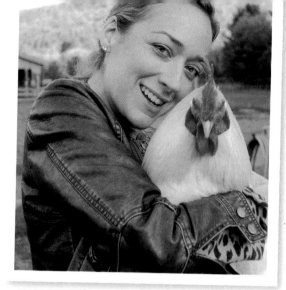

When rain forest is killed, it stops breathing and atmospheric CO_2 levels rise. This is also true of our oceans, the other great carbon sink. Coral reefs are like underwater rain forests, teeming with biodiversity. They, too, are endangered as more and more of them die in acidic dead zones.

In 2008 Dr. Rajendra Pachauri, the chair of the prestigious United Nations Intergovernmental Panel on Climate Change (IPCC), made waves when he said that reducing meat consumption was the most immediate way to take action against global warming. He suggested we "Give up meat for one day [per week] initially and decrease it from there." In 2010 the UN further upped the ante by urging a global move towards a meat- and dairy-free diet: "A vegan diet is vital to save the world from hunger, fuel poverty, and the worst impacts of climate change." Let's face it, ladies—one day a week without meat? You can do it with your eyes closed. How about three days a week, or five, or seven?

It's understandable why quality food is condemned as elitist, and why many people, especially the poor, buy cheap food. But now you can see how the 99-cent burger doesn't really cost 99 cents. There's always more to a story than meets the eye, and it's especially true with our way of eating.

A DAY IN THE LIFE of a FACTORY FARM *with Wayne Pacelle*

The cruelties of factory farming, with its intensive animal confinement practices and well-documented transport and slaughter abuses, have come to the public's attention in an unprecedented manner in recent years. Now there is a clamor for reform. By passing laws in a number of states to ban small crates and cages that do not allow the animals to engage in even the most basic movement, working to pass a comprehensive federal ban on the mistreatment and slaughter of downed cattle, and successfully working with corporations to expand their vegan options and improve animal welfare in their supply chains, the animal protection movement is advancing the argument that eating is a moral act and that Americans cannot sidestep the problems spawned by modern-day industrial animal agribusiness.

Why the fuss about how we treat farm animals? Quite simply, because some standard agribusiness practices are now demonstrably out of step with mainstream American values about how animals ought to be treated. The fifty-year experiment with factory farming has been successful in terms of producing vast quantities of meat, milk, and eggs at a cheap price point, but it has failed to calculate the broader costs of the enterprise—extreme animal suffering, air and water pollution, and serious public health threats, including the reckless overuse of antibiotics and the potential for the emergence of antibiotic-resistant bacteria.

Polls show that Americans overwhelmingly favor ending the extreme confinement of farm animals, and when given the chance to take action, voters favor reform time and again. Yet

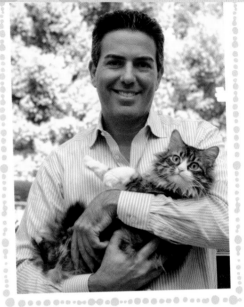

Michelle Riley/The HSUS

animal agribusinesses persist in subjecting farm animals to abuses that would warrant criminal cruelty prosecution if the animals were dogs or cats. For example, US egg factory farms confine close to 280 million egg-laying hens into barren battery cages for the bulk of their lives—up to eighteen months. Crowded into these wire cages, they cannot even spread their wings, let alone nest, dust-bathe, perch, or walk more than a step or so. Each bird has less space than a sheet of letter-size paper on which to live for a year before she's slaughtered. Animals built to move should be allowed to move, and it's just not fair to subject them to this privation.

Similarly, hundreds of thousands of veal calves across the United States are forced into crates too narrow for them to turn around or lie down comfortably. Typically chained by their necks, they're virtually immobilized and can't engage in natural behaviors.

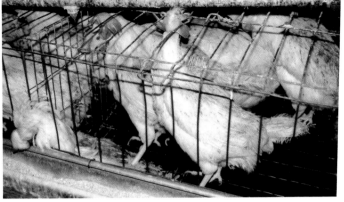

Overcrowded chickens

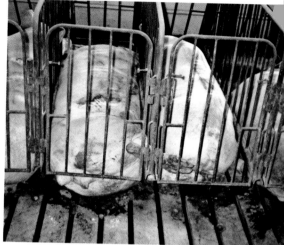

Pigs in gestation crates

Our nation's factory farms confine millions of breeding pigs in gestation crates—2-foot-wide individual metal cages barely bigger than their bodies—for nearly their entire four-month pregnancies. These intelligent, sociable animals suffer terribly, and they develop crippling joint disorders and lameness from the cramped conditions.

There are other practices in industrial agriculture that violate our basic values about proper care of animals. Foie gras producers force-feed ducks and geese so severely that the animals' livers swell to ten times their normal size, inducing a disease state as a normal production practice. Chickens and turkeys constitute 95 percent of all animals slaughtered for food in America, yet the USDA exempts them from the minimal standards of the Humane Methods of Slaughter Act.

Despite industry claims that it adheres to humane practices, we've seen a steady stream of undercover investigations pull the curtain back on sickening and unacceptable abuses: In California, downed cows tormented to get them to stand. In Ohio, pigs killed by execution-style hanging. Turkeys kicked, punched, and stomped on in West Virginia. Pigs beaten with blunt instruments in North Carolina. Egg-laying hens thrown into trash cans to die a slow, painful

death in Maine. Still more egg-laying hens impaled on cage wires in California.

Of course, it's not only common sense that says such abuse is wrong. Independent science on animal welfare also buttresses the case for reform. For example, the prestigious Pew Commission on Industrial Farm Animal Production—a disinterested panel that included former Kansas governor John Carlin, former US secretary of agriculture Dan Glickman, farm animal researchers, veterinarians, and ranchers—extensively studied the issue for two and a half years. The commissioners reviewed the body of scientific literature on the topic and unanimously concluded that battery cages, gestation crates, and veal crates should be phased out.

Concern about animal welfare is ascendant. If current trends are an indicator, cultural and political circumstances are breaking in the direction of concern for farm animals. When I became vegan in 1985, finding vegan food was a chore and the term itself was, to say the least, unfamiliar. Today it's part of the American lexicon, and supermarkets, restaurants, and other food outlets often offer vegan fare. Books like *Skinny Bitch* and *The Engine 2 Diet* enjoy a vast popular audience, especially with young people, and especially girls and women.

Nearly four hundred universities have opted to switch some or all of their egg purchasing away from battery cage operators. And an increasing number of major retailers are moving away from the most abusive animal products, like foie gras and battery cage eggs.

While just a decade ago our movement was in a preregulation period with regard to farm animal welfare, there's been steady progress in the direction of reform. Arizona, Colorado, Florida, Maine, and Oregon have passed laws, either through state legislatures or citizen initiatives, phasing out certain kinds of intensive confinement.

In a November 2008 election, California voters passed in a landslide vote the Prevention of Farm Animal Cruelty Act, which phases out battery cages, veal crates, and gestation crates. It was the most popular citizen ballot initiative in California's history, attracting nearly 64 percent of the vote and a raft of media attention—exposure that further embeds the idea of farm animal welfare into the public consciousness.

There is no more important thing we can do for animals than start conscious eating. With 10 billion animals raised for food, it is the biggest form of animal use of all. From World War II until very recently, the situation has grown increasingly harsh for animals, and it's just now starting to turn around. We all need to be part of the solution. Don't leave it up to anyone else. You have the power to help animals, and also to spread the word, urging others to abstain from eating meat, eggs, and dairy, to reduce intake of animal products, or at least to stop purchasing products from factory farms. All animals deserve respect and moral consideration, including farm animals.

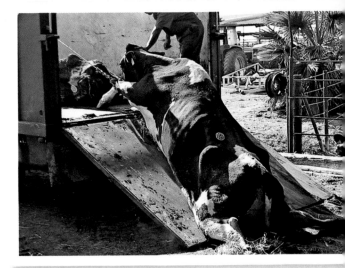

Downer cows on the the their way to slaughter

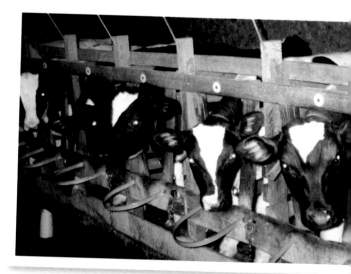

Veal calves

Wayne Pacelle is president and CEO of the Humane Society of the United States. He is cofounder and former chairman of Humane USA, a nonpartisan organization that works to elect humane-minded candidates to political office.

Photos courtesy of Farm Sanctuary and the Humane Society

MAKE THE CONNECTION

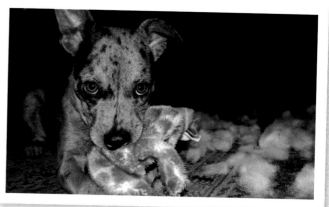

Lola, rescued a day before scheduled euthanization

Ninety-nine percent of the animal products we consume come from factory farms. I know it's hard to look at these horrors. Paul McCartney once said, "If slaughterhouses had glass walls, everyone would be a vegetarian."

Today some farmers are following more sustainable methods of raising beef cattle, poultry and other Beings. They treat their animals more humanely (though they still end up at the same slaughterhouses). Their meat is very expensive, easily three times or more costly than industrial raised flesh. Small farms, like the one I grew up next to, don't receive government subsidies. You're paying for healthy livestock without the dangerous shortcuts and drugs.

If after all you've learned, you still want to include some meat and dairy in your diet, research a local organic producer. Keep in mind that just because the label says "free range," "organic," "natural," or "grass-fed" doesn't mean the animals were treated well. If suffering matters to you, limit the amount of nonindustrial animals you eat or buy meat with the Certified Humane Raised and Handled food label. It's the only program in the United States dedicated to improving the welfare of farm animals from birth through slaughter.

Perhaps you're still having a hard time with these issues. You may even be angry or agitated at the suggestion to consider animal welfare when preparing your dinner. The compassion lightbulb really turned on for me when I thought about our dog Lola (the best rescue pooch ever!). She has a Christmas stocking. Lola knows more words than some of the kids I taught at NYU. Pigs are no less intelligent, emotional, or social creatures. Calves are sensitive and playful. Chickens love to gossip with their friends. And all mothers love their babies. Let's take feminism to the next level and stand beside *all* our sisters, including those with fur and feathers. If we could make the connection between our pets and our plates, we'd respect these Beings more. At the very least, we would demand better conditions for them, and we would grant them a swift and painless death.

The aforementioned Meatless Monday campaign, in association with the Johns Hopkins School of Public Health, provides lots of recipes, nutritional guidelines, and cooking tips on the Web site www.meatlessmonday.com. Just remember the Crazy Sexy pH nuggets you learned in chapter 2 and stack your plate with more alkaline chow.

My brilliant friend Kathy Freston has this advice for folks who can't bear to live without certain meaty pleasures: "If you just can't give up one particular animal product, that's okay. Give up all of the other ones instead. A friend told me that he loves burgers too much to give them up; I suggested that he give up all animal products except burgers. Some of my friends can't give up ice cream or cream in their coffee or whatever—so give up everything but that. That's a huge step forward, and I suspect that after eating mostly vegetarian for a while, you'll decide that those burgers or that ice cream aren't so tasty anymore."

SOY AS A MEAT PROTEIN SUBSTITUTE

There are lots of meat stand-ins on the market today, many of which are made from beans, grains, and veggies, and especially soy. However, you'll notice that when I talk about soy consumption, I generally accompany my recommendations with the words *in moderation.* Studies in Asian communities show that the health benefits of soy come from condiment-size portions of fermented soy foods. While soy is high in protein (in fact, it's a complete protein), tastes yummy, and is less expensive than meat, most of the soy we eat is processed, genetically modified, heavily sprayed, and supersized. As much as possible, eat soy in its natural form.

Choice one: Soybeans and edamame. If you consume tofu, keep it to small amounts and buy organic brands (you can even find sprouted varieties).

Choice two: Fermented soy—tempeh, natto, and miso. Fermented foods have a probiotic effect and are the easiest forms for your body to digest and absorb. The fermentation process also helps to neutralize the high levels of phytic acids (which may block the absorption of minerals like calcium, magnesium, zinc, and iron). See chapter 8 for more info about fabulous fermented goodies.

Because there's lots of disagreement among doctors and researchers about whether soy is God or the devil, I'm not going to claim to have the answers. Some researchers believe that soy foods increase bone density and even stave off hot flashes. They claim that the isoflavones found in soy can help prevent breast cancer or keep it from recurring. But if you already have breast cancer, particularly if it's the estrogen-sensitive kind, those same isoflavones could promote the growth of the disease. Ditto for uterine and ovarian cancer, which are also estrogen-sensitive. And for you guys, there's some evidence that the hormonal effects of soy can promote prostate cancer. Isoflavones can also create potential thyroid complications and mess with endocrine function.

Soy is definitely the ball in a game of contradictory-research Ping-Pong. But here's what I know for sure: The more processed the soy product, the worse it is for you. I'm talking about faux meats, treats, and snacks. Processed soy is acidic and mucus-forming. Though it's a helpful transition food as you move toward a vegetarian or vegan diet, don't overdo it. Also, stick with organic brands.

DON'T HAVE A COW!

Wow—I know this chapter was a biggie. As you feel better, look better, and smile brighter, you will naturally continue to lean toward a healthier way of eating. You'll want more greens and less flesh. Remember, one of the principles of the Crazy Sexy Diet is balancing the pH of your body. If occasionally eating small amounts of non-factory-farmed animal products keeps you on track, fine. But the more you eat, the more inflamed and acidic you will become. And the money you save by not buying meat can be put toward organic vegetables, a class that excites you, or a relaxing beach vacation!

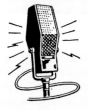

testimonial: Maria M.

At twenty years old I was running for a division one university. I began experiencing some unusual pain in both of my legs. Three years later, when I could no longer stand up for more than a few minutes, I was diagnosed with Reflex Sympathetic Dystrophy. At that point the pain had spread from both feet to almost every inch of my body and I was staring a wheelchair in the face. In my desperation for the pain to end, I signed up for an experimental five-day inpatient IV ketamine infusion. A day before I headed into NYC to have this experimental procedure done, I went to Best Buy to find a neat documentary to watch in the hospital. I came across *Crazy Sexy Cancer*, and my whole life changed! Obviously, the procedure did not work, and it was awful! When I was discharged, my parents bought me a juicer, and I have never looked back. I took matters into my own hands and changed my diet, incorporated meditation, prayer, and other spiritual practices including yoga. A year after my diagnosis, I am healthier than I have ever been, even with this disease. With this lifestyle as a supplement to my pain medications, I have avoided a wheelchair and received a 4.0 GPA in my first year of graduate school (for social work). I am by far beating the odds. Thank you, Kris!!!!

CHAPTER 4 IN REVIEW

REMEMBER:

- You can get all the protein and calcium you need from a varied plant-based diet.

- That same plant-based diet is the best prevention against heart disease, cancer, and diabetes.

- Dairy causes mucus buildup and has been linked to a variety of illnesses, from asthma to arthritis to Crohn's disease.

- Processed meats are big-time no-nos: salt, fat, body parts, and carcinogens.

- Behind every pound of meat sold lies a cascade of hidden costs to our health, economy, and environment.

- Try weaning yourself off animal products. Start slow (cut them out one day per week), then build up to more days.

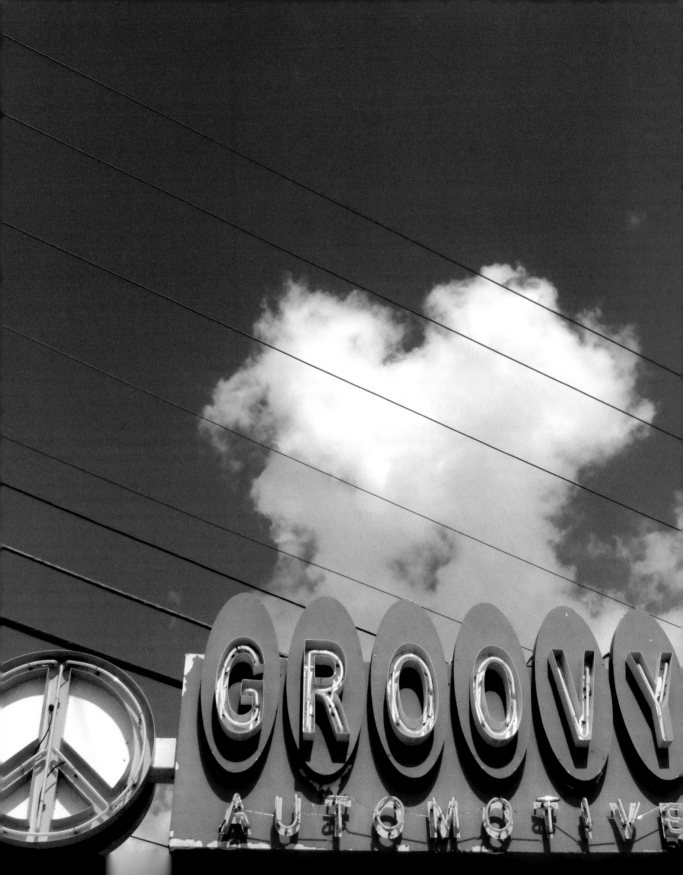

GO WITH YOUR
GUT

You've heard it a million times: You are what you eat. 'Tis true, and my twist on this old saw takes it a step farther: You're also what you don't poop. If you're haulin' around garbage in your cells, tissues, or colon, you're literally waste-ing your vibrant potential. Ideally, healthy real food goes in, contributes to the cause (you), and comes out in an effortless and timely fashion. Sadly, this isn't the case for the majority of Americans.

Unhealthy food clogs all aspects of your God pod, screws up your immune system, stages a bacterial coup, and creates a biohazardous environment. Yet another reason why the alkaline, energy-packed foods on the Crazy Sexy Diet can help you heal. In this chapter you'll learn the importance of your majestic root system—your digestion. Warning: We're gonna talk shit. It's time to stop being lady-like, start farting with pride, and examine what does and doesn't come out of your ass. Your health depends on it.

A TOUR OF YOUR DIGESTION

When I was a kid, I used to love to watch a show called *The Love Boat* with my grandma. We both adored cruise director Julie McCoy, and I dreamed of having a job like hers when I grew up. Grandma would join me and off we'd sail to Fantasy Island to dine with Mr. Roarke and Tattoo. Little did I know that the tour I'd be giving would be very different from a high-seas expedition. So indulge my childhood dreams, and allow me to be the Julie McCoy of digestion.

Digestion is the process of extracting nutrients from food and preparing the leftover waste for elimination from the body. It starts in your mouth and finishes, or so you hope, with a soft-serve plop in your royal commode. The whole system is basically one long twisting, turning tube of biochemical fun.

Your mouth is the first stop on the cruise. As you chew, enzymes in your saliva begin to break down your food. Next, the chunks of chow voyage to your tummy (après swallowing), where they churn and mix with hydrochloric acid and other gastric juices until all is transformed into a substance called chyme.

Once the food (chyme) leaves your tummy, it enters your small intestine, where additional enzymes and digestive juices break it down further.

Your small intestine is also the sweet spot where the nutrients are absorbed into your body. Next stop, your large intestine, also known as your colon. What's left after absorption is mostly fiber, undigested food bits, dead bacteria, digestive juices, and water. Your large intestine's job is to reabsorb most of the remaining water and turn the leftover chyme into poop.

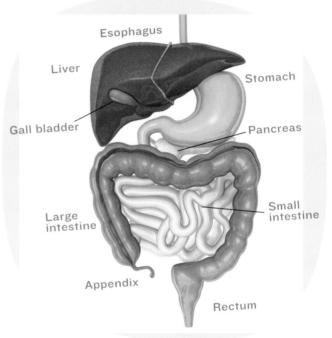

Esophagus
Liver
Stomach
Gall bladder
Pancreas
Large intestine
Small intestine
Appendix
Rectum

TAKE OUT THE TRASH

Be honest, do you poop on a regular basis? Like after each meal or at least once per day? If you aren't having abundant bowel movements on a daily basis, then you're full of shit, lady. There may be days', even weeks' worth of debris just hanging

out and backing you up. No matter how healthy our diets, if our inner sewer system is clogged, our bodies break down. Many of us have impacted and encrusted colons from years of eating excess meat, dairy, processed foods, breads, candies, cookies, bad oils, and other tasty (but toxic) treats.

Did you know that the average person might be hauling around between 7 and 10 extra pounds just in the colon? Gross! Medical autopsy lore has it that Elvis was carrying about 60 pounds of poo and fried peanut butter/banana sandwiches up his ass when he expired. While I doubt that's true, extra pounds are possible, and here's why. Your intestines are about 26 feet long. If you were to spread them out, their surface—includ-

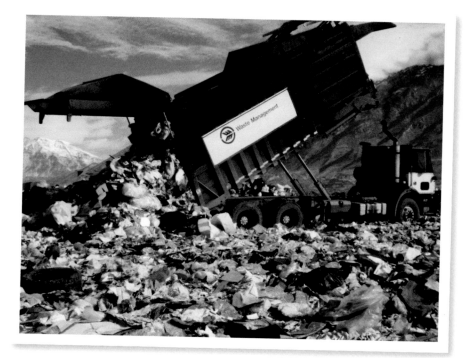

ing all the nooks, crannies and intestinal villi—would cover a tennis court. With that in mind, you can imagine countless hiding places for waste to get trapped.

Lining the walls of the small intestine are millions of tiny, finger-like protrusions called villi. They expand the total surface of the small intestine so that you can absorb more nutrients. When food passes over the villi, they draw in nutrients. But if they're damaged, the nutrients just cruise on by.

If waste doesn't move steadily through the colon, it stagnates, rots, and hardens, causing myriad problems, such as constipation, upset stomach and cramping, a weakened immune system, weight gain, and even depression.

It stands to reason, then, that if our inner sewer system is clogged, our bodies break down. Your immune system relies greatly on your intestines. In fact, 60 to 70 percent of your immune power is in your digestive tract, starting with lymphatic tissue in your tonsils and ending in your rectum. Like a warrior

princess, your immune system kills off any bad germs and parasites that you lick up in your food.

You carry around literally trillions of bacteria in your intestines. Generally speaking, they're friendly little guys who busily help you digest your food and even make some vitamins, like vitamin K. You also carry around plenty of not-so-friendly bacteria, such as one called *Clostridium difficile* that can even kill people with weakened immune systems. Usually the good guys crowd out the bad, but if the bad guys get enough of a foothold to multiply then they can cause real problems.

That's the theory, anyway. In fact, lots of things can mess up your intestinal bacteria and the friendly bacteria you depend on for good health. Top of the list? Poor diet—especially too much sugar, too much animal protein, and too little fiber. Also on the list are drugs, especially antibiotics and alcohol.

Some doctors, nutritionists, and now advertisers suggest yogurt as a means of getting some extra good bacteria, also known as probiotics, into your system (I'll explain a lot more about this in chapter 9). But given what we've learned about dairy products (and pasteurization), this advice is far from sound. Remember, milk creates mucus, and mucus creates inflammation, stagnation, and a whole lotta disorder in your gut. In addition, most yogurts are loaded with added sugar. Bad bacteria love to feed and multiply on sugar. And don't be fooled into buying a vat of ice cream called yogurt. As you've learned, most health claims have been manufactured in boardrooms. What you're really getting is a ton of empty calories, lots of fat, sugar, and mucus.

SHIT FOR BRAINS

Ever heard of the brain–gut connection? Dr. Michael Gershon, a researcher at Columbia University, calls the gut the "second brain." The gut has its very own nervous system—the small intestine alone has as many neurons as your spinal cord. Neurotransmitters are natural chemicals that transmit signals from one part of your brain to another. Guess what? They're also found in your intestines. In fact, a whopping 95 percent of all serotonin, one of the most important neurotransmitters, is made by nerve cells in your gut. And get this—the gut has at least seven different kinds of serotonin receptors. An imbalance in serotonin levels can be an underlying cause of depression. If one brain is out of balance, it stands to reason that the other one (the one you're using to read this) might be out of balance, too. Many people with depression and anxiety also have bowel trouble. Maybe we need to pop less Prozac and pump out more poop.

THE SLIME OF YOUR LIFE

Mucus. It sounds pretty disgusting, but this slippery goo serves a very necessary protective function in the body. Mucus membranes are located throughout your body, not just in the booger factory. In fact, humans produce about a liter of it a day. Mucus guards your stomach lining from hydrochloric acid, helps prevent infection in your cervix, and protects you from what your body senses as foreign invaders. A small amount of mucus in your intestines lubes the tubes in order to move waste through smoothly. However, a daily onslaught of bad eating habits creates excess mucus and problems like constipation. We all know what it's like to have a congested, dripping nose. Well, imagine your nose is your colon (gross, I know, just go with it). Try pushing a poop through all the goo.

As you've already learned, mucus is also acidic. Too much of it lowers our pH and reduces our oxygen levels. Next step, inflammation, which does what? Creates more mucus! It becomes a vicious cycle of inner snot. Yuck. After years of poor dietary habits, antibiotics, drugs, and stimulants, many people are surprised at the endless amount of mucus that pours from their bodies. In *The Mucusless Diet Healing System,* Arnold Ehret writes, "All disease is a result of constitutional constipation. The entire human pipe system is chronically constipated through the wrong foods of civilization."

In order to cleanse properly, you need a break from the bad food and toxins that go in your body, as well as help moving the old crud out. This is why I combine an optional one-day green juice fast and colon hydrotherapy as part of my 21-Day Cleanse

(see chapter 10). During the detox process, even more trash than usual is dumped into the colon and bloodstream, so it's extra important to keep moving the waste out. Once you've given your terrain a spring cleaning and upgraded your diet Crazy Sexy style, you'll only need to cleanse occasionally. Until then, read on.

A daily onslaught of bad eating habits creates excess mucus and problems like constipation.

UNCLOG YOUR PIPES WITH AN INNER PLUMBER

Imagine an old house that's been locked up for decades, inhabited by reclusive socialite wackadoos like the Beales in *Grey Gardens.* When you start sweeping, you awaken a dust storm. If you don't open the windows, the dirt just relocates. The same holds true for your God pod. One of the best ways to keep the dust from settling in your inner house is with an internal bath that moves the junk out the back door: an enema or colonic.

Lots of folks get squirmy or prudish at the mention of poop—especially when it also involves putting something up their butt. "That's unnatural! Stuff goes out, you don't stick it in!" Well, get over it. PowerBars are unnatural, cleansing is not. Colon cleansing is a healing method that has been used since the ancient Egyptians. Well into the 1900s, enemas were widely administered by community doctors. In fact, they have long been considered one of the best remedies for a headache! When your system stalls and sputters from the Standard American Diet, colon

hydrotherapy may well be in order. It's much more effective and gentle than harsh, habit-forming chemical laxatives such as Ex-Lax or even herbal laxatives containing senna. Laxatives also irritate and further weaken the colon and can cause dehydration. If you're not evacuating on a regular basis or if you're about to embark on a cleanse, you should definitely consider the power of the hose.

THE ABCS OF ENEMAS

Enemas help get the lower part of the colon, called the descending colon, moving and grooving. They are easy to administer at home and can provide much relief for those who suffer from constipation. Step one for using an enema: Make peace with the fact that you're gonna put a helpful hose up your ass. Step two: Deck out your bathroom like a detox ashram. Just because said hose is up your ass doesn't mean you have to be in an antiseptic environment. Surround yourself with style and beauty.

I like to roll out my yoga mat and then place a big comfy towel on top. Turn down the lights, play some music, light a candle, and relax.

Most enema bags come in 1- or 2-quart sizes and require you to fasten the tube to the bag. No problemo—when filling the bag, make sure the clamp on the tube is in the closed position, otherwise the water will flood your ashram, not your ass. Fill the enema bag with lukewarm filtered or distilled water. (Chlorine in tap water kills the good flora in your colon.) Before inserting the tube in your tush, let a little water out of the enema into the sink—this removes air bubbles. Next, hang the enema bag on a towel rack or doorknob, making sure that the bag is higher than you (gravity rocks!). Lie on your left side with your right knee bent close to your chest, left leg straight. Lubricate the tube tip with a bit of coconut oil and then gently insert the tube into your rectum. Woo hoo! Ya don't need to go far, Rambo—2 to 3 inches will do.

Release the clamp and let the water begin to fill you slowly. If you let too much water in too fast, you may get an urge to evacuate prematurely. For the best results, you'll want to fill for a bit, then clamp off and relax, allowing the water to create a soaking cycle. When you feel ready, let more water in. If you're feeling adventurous, roll slowly onto your back with your knees bent and begin to massage your belly, moving clockwise. This is best done during a soaking cycle.

Next, roll slowly onto your right side, allowing the water to hit other areas. Wild women may want to try the kneeling position. Wha? Place your head on the floor and kneel, as if creating a tripod. Just make sure your door is locked and your ass is facing the other direction!

Finish up by clamping off the tube and slowly removing the tip. Try to hold the water for fifteen to twenty minutes, and then let it all go into the toilet bowl. If you can't hold it for that long, no

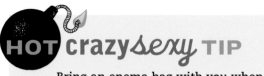

worries—let it go when you're ready. Feel free to do another round if you didn't release much the first time. Sometimes gas is the main thing in the way; once that's removed you'll have a better round two. If you get bored, bring a book or a recorded inspirational lecture. Perhaps you'll hold the water longer if you put your focus on Deepak Chopra. When you're finished, empty the bag of any remaining water and send some hot water through to flush it. Wash with mild organic soap and water. To avoid passing germs around, here's a party tip: Don't share your enema bag with anyone—duh!

GRASS UP YOUR ASS

Wheatgrass is just what it sounds like: the young shoots put up by sprouting wheat seeds. Wheatgrass is a powerful tonic for healing through both drinking (see chapter 6) and as a sidekick to your enema. One 4-ounce shot made at home or bought fresh from the juice bar is like hooking your immune system up to a set of jumper cables. An implant is a small amount of juice held in the lower bowel for about twenty minutes. In the case of illness, wheatgrass implants stimulate a rapid cleansing and healing of the lower bowel. Implants also help to draw out accumulated debris. This stimulates peristalsis and replenishes the electrolytes in your colon.

Colon hydrotherapy with a wheatgrass chaser is also a good deal for the big daddy of all organs—your liver. Once implanted, a portion of the juice is absorbed into the hepatic vein, which travels directly to the liver. The juice stimulates your liver to purge and gives it a great boost of the mighty healer chlorophyll (think oxygen).

Your liver is really the chief organ of elimination. Think of it as the body's recycling center, constantly filtering and cleaning the blood. The liver also plays a vital role in digestion, assimilation, your immune system, and literally hundreds of other processes. It's one busy dude! Once it gets clogged, so do you.

HIGH ON COLONICS

Colonics are even better than enemas (I know, you're thinking nothing could be better than an enema!) because they can access the entire colon: ascending, transverse, and descending. A colonic machine uses very gentle water pressure to introduce the water deep into the colon. While an enema uses only about 1 quart of water, a colonic can use up to 6 gallons over the course of the treatment. As you can imagine, colonics are not DIY projects—you need a trained professional.

An average session with a colon therapist lasts from forty-five minutes to an hour. If you're really backed up or if you have health issues that would benefit from deeper detoxification, you may have to do a series of treatments in the beginning. The number of treatments you'll need really depends on the condition of your health and your colon—a good therapist will tell you where you stand.

If you've never had a colonic, the first time can be very intimidating. There is absolutely nothing to worry about. You won't poop on the table or squirt water across the room. In fact, it's all very sanitary and matter-of-fact. There are two types of colonics, gravity and pressurized. An expert hydrotherapist can do wonders with either method, but I recommend gravity colonics, since pressurized units can actually cause more impaction if you're already really blocked up. Gravity units use only the force

of gravity (like an enema, but bigger) to control water flow, so they're gentler, especially for people with sensitive GI tracts or IBS. The therapist gently inserts the lubricated speculum into your rectum while you're covered with a towel or sheet from the waist down. The water is slowly introduced—"Well, hello there, water"—then you fill and soak much as you do with an enema.

As you soak, a lovely belly rub is gently administered. A good therapist knows how to access pressure points on your calves, feet, and back that will help you expel poo materials. When you're ready to release, the flow is reversed and the water and waste depart from the same tube. It's a completely closed system, so that means there's no muss, no fuss, and no odor. You can even see what's headed to pasture through a little viewing window in the machine. Now, that's cool! Some therapists are like mystical tea-leaf-reading psychics! One look at your poop and they've got you figured out. You'll learn a lot about what is and what isn't working with your digestion. More than likely you'll witness lots of mucus, gas bubbles, bile, undigested food ("When did I eat corn?"), and maybe some parasites cruisin' by. Sometimes it's better than a trip to the zoo!

Folks who oppose colon therapy claim you can become dependent on it. This isn't really a worry. Think of colon therapy like a workout: The gentle pressure from the water actually tones and rebuilds your muscles by making peristalsis—the contraction of smooth muscles that propels stuff through the digestive tract—stronger. Once the initial cleansing process is complete, colonics need only be used for maintenance and upkeep once per season or a couple of times a year.

Another criticism is that colon therapy washes away good bacteria. In fact, good bacteria can only breed in a clean environment. A probiotic (see chapter 9) can be taken after cleansing to help repopulate the colon with good bacteria. The colon will rebalance itself with a better ratio of friendly to unfriendly bacteria, especially when all the debris is cleared away.

The one real concern you should have about colon therapy is the cleanliness of the provider. Colon therapists don't have to be licensed or certified—pretty much anyone can buy a machine and go into practice. To avoid unskilled or inexperienced practitioners or those who might be careless about sanitation, get a personal recommendation if possible. Ask around among the people in your community who are most likely to know: chiropractors, massage therapists, naturopaths, nutritionists. Ask for and check references! My resource section on crazysexylife.com also lists several national databases.

Be prepared for some crazy (not so) sexy purging. If your diet is mildly bad, then your detox will be mildly uncomfortable. If your diet resembles a

HOT crazysexy TIP

If you are pregnant; suffering from a flare-up of Crohn's disease, irritable bowel syndrome, or acute diverticulitis; if you're having diarrhea; or if you've ever had any portion of your colon removed, then colonics are not advised.

train wreck, then hang on tight, 'cause it's gonna be a bumpy ride, baby! Just remember, this too shall pass (that's the point). It's better to get the crap out with an enema or colonic than to let it pile up and wage a secret war on your insides. For now, know that most symptoms you feel during the process are totally normal and harmless. Desperate times call for deeper cleaning.

DETOXING YOUR BODY
with Alejandro Junger, MD

Detoxification is as necessary for life as the beating of the heart. Our cells are constantly forming toxins as normal waste products of metabolism. The cells release the toxins into the blood; within a few heartbeats, the toxins are swept into the liver for detoxification.

The detoxification process is amazingly intricate. While the toxins are still in your bloodstream, circulating antioxidants latch onto them, neutralize their oxidizing capacity, and escort them to the liver. Once there, a liver cell grabs onto the toxin and releases the antioxidant molecule to go back into circulation. The liver cell then gets to work on the toxin.

Detoxification processing has two steps. In phase 1 chemical reactions within the liver neutralize and then eliminate the toxin by one of three routes:

- Sending it into the bile to eventually pass out of the body in feces.
- Sending it into the urine and sweat to be eliminated that way.
- Converting it into an intermediate compound that may actually be more toxic than the original toxin.

When a toxin is converted, phase 2 detoxification kicks in to deal with the intermediate compounds. During this process, additional chemical reactions in the liver neutralize the compound and make it water-soluble. Once that process is complete, the neutralized toxin can be eliminated through the urine or sweat.

All the complex chemical detoxification reactions in the liver are made possible by a group of enzymes known as the cytochrome p450 series. To function properly, these enzymes need plenty of nutrients such as vitamin C, the B vitamins, selenium, magnesium, sulfur, and amino acids like methionine and cysteine.

Evolution has designed your detox system to handle a natural diet that's high in fresh, raw, and alkalizing plant foods. If we humans ate just our natural diet, we would have all the antioxidants we need to protect our bodies from the oxidative damage caused by circulating toxins. We'd also have in abundance all the nutrients the liver needs to perform phase 1 and 2 detoxification efficiently.

So intricate, intelligent, and predictive is nature's design that it has built-in backup mechanisms in case of excess toxicity. Since the most likely situation if any toxin accumulates is acidity, the body can turn on one or more backup systems to restore the pH balance. Breathing faster releases more carbon dioxide, an acid; this is one way your body can compensate, at least for a short time, for a sudden rise in acidity. If the acidity is persistent, your body will release calcium and other minerals from your bones to neutralize it. This fizzling of the bones means they are literally dissolving themselves. Down the line comes osteoporosis.

Nature has included backup systems because acid overload has always been a possibility. Those backup systems are designed to work only now and then, because they shouldn't be needed more than now and then. In the past few hundred years, however, the human diet has shifted into a red zone that constantly calls on our backup systems.

Here's what happened:

Modern life has added thousands of toxins to the picture. Foods today are loaded with chemicals and heavily processed. Instead of eating actual nutrients, we digest food-like molecules that trick the body into absorbing them. Once inside the body, they can't be used. Within the body, they cause irritation and inflammation; in the liver, phase 1 metabolization turns them into even worse poisons. In addition to the coloring agents, fragrance agents, texturizing agents, and artificial flavoring, we also ingest toxic chemicals such as hormones that can interfere with our body's signaling.

Our overall environment also has seen an exponential increase in the amount and variety of chemicals that are not naturally occurring— they're concocted in a laboratory. The air we breathe, the water we wash with and drink, the cosmetics we use, the laundry detergents, the paint on our walls, the fire retardant off-gassing from the mattress . . .

Because of our constant exposure to chemicals, our intestinal flora—the bacteria we depend on for good health—are in danger of extinction. They're under massive direct and indirect attack. Direct attack happens when we take antibiotics. Indirect attacks happen because we're constantly exposed to antibacterial agents. Preservatives, conservatives, pesticides, insecticides, antibacterials, antivirals—we're exposed to them every time we wash or clean our bodies, our clothing, our homes, our workplaces. Even some toys for children have antibacterial products built in to them. Killing off our intestinal flora is knocking over the first domino that ends up manifesting as many of the chronic diseases that became epidemics.

Nutrients are becoming scarce even as the quantity of food explodes. Depleted soils, farming practices, transportation, irradiation, pasteurization, not chewing thoroughly, and the death of the intestinal flora—all make it almost impossible to end up with enough nutrients from the diet for a harmonious metabolism and vibrant health. At the same time, nutrient depletion turns on hunger sensations. Your body wants and needs those nutrients, and the only way it knows to get them is to make you feel hungry so you'll eat more. Only when your body detects that the needed nutrients have been consumed will the hunger stop. But if your food never really gives you those nutrients in adequate amounts and in forms your body can use, you never stop feeling hungry.

In summary, in modern life you're exposed to more toxins than your body is designed to handle. Your body has to work much harder to eliminate them, while also coping with a lack of good intestinal bacteria and a shortage of nutrients. This is an evolutionary glitch—your body can't evolve fast enough to handle our modern diet. What to do instead? Return your diet—and your body—to the way of eating it is designed for. That means lots of raw and lightly cooked foods and regular elimination. Avoid adding toxins to your body by avoiding added poisons from cleaning supplies, antibiotics, and other chemically laden products. Clean versions that are better for you and the planet are readily available.

Alejandro Junger, MD, is the best-selling author of *Clean: The Revolutionary Program to Restore the Body's Natural Ability to Heal Itself.*

SQUATTER'S RIGHTS

There are three times in life when squatting is necessary. One: childbirth. Two: if you're employed as an umpire. Three: dropping the kids off at the pool, aka taking a crap. The modern can just wasn't designed in your colon's best interest. Ideally, your feet should be elevated about 10 to 18 inches off the ground—you want your knees to be higher than your hips.

I'll never forget the first time I saw a squat toilet while working in a rural area of Japan. Basically, it's a hole in the ground with a flusher. I thought, You've got to be kidding. When I asked my interpreter why the toilets in town were so freaky, he laughed and said, "It's your toilets that are freaky, my dear." Hmmm. Many years later, while studying the colon, I realized my Japanese host was right. The squatting position is the way we're naturally designed for pooping. By raising your feet to simulate a squat position, you encourage ("that-a-girl!") a complete removal of waste.

No need to ask your plumber to take out your toilet and install a hole in your bathroom. Renewlife.com sells a LifeSTEP support stool that fits around your toilet so that your feet can rest in the anatomically correct position for healthy elimination. You can find a fancier version (a bit more chic and attractive) at miraclestep.com. If you want to be thrifty, just use a small hamper or trash can—that's what I use. In addition to squatting, strong abdominals really help move things along. Do your sit-ups, folks! Happy pooping!

FOOD COMBINING

Another way to create optimum digestion, assimilation, and elimination for better energy and overall health is strategic food combining. Different foods have different transit schedules (the time it takes from entry to exit) and require different digestive enzymes and varying acid/alkaline conditions. When we combine food properly, we can manage the traffic in our gut to move smoothly and without jams. When we don't, the resulting gridlock creates road rage. The result? Foul farts, rot, too much mucus, constipation, partly digested food in your commode, and bloating that makes you blame your nice trousers.

Not everyone is sensitive to dense, miscombined meals. Perhaps you have the constitution of a gladiator and this step will only make you feel restricted and pissed. If so, forget it! Food combining is a somewhat new concept, and while there are many respected health practitioners who swear by its value, others think it's a lot of nonsense. Be a curious Wellness Warrior and try it for yourself. If you suffer from belly and bowel troubles after meals, you may see a big difference. My guess is that you won't have to experiment for long. A few days to a week should be enough to know if food combining is helping you.

When I teach nutrition classes in my workshops, I usually bring a fancy lace bra and a pair of my husband's paint-stained overalls to explain the principles of food combining. Picture those filthy work pants covered in grease, paint, and God only knows what else in your washer. Those stank pants need to be soaked and laundered in boiling hot water with lots of Seventh Generation detergent and maybe a splash of natural bleach.

The metal clasps make loud banging noises and nothing but rags are safe with them in the spin

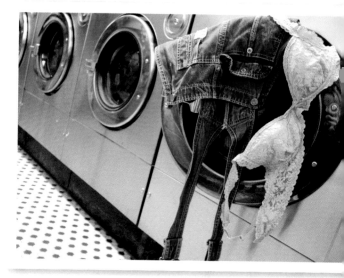

cycle. Would you put your lovely (and extremely expensive) La Perla bra in the wash with that brute? My guess is no. If you did, your lady holders would be torn to shreds and useless. Tit slings need the delicate cycle. Dirty dog pants need a power shower. If you put them in the delicate cycle, they will remain filthy. Get the picture? Your bra and his pants require different transit times to get clean and spiffy.

Different foods have different transit schedules (the time it takes from entry to exit) and require different digestive enzymes and varying acid/alkaline conditions.

COMBO BASICS

The basic principles of food combining are pretty simple. Here's a list to get you started. To see these principles in action, check out Monday in my "Crazy Sexy Day in the Life" portion of chapter 10.

- Eat melon alone or leave it alone (fifteen to thirty minutes' digestion time).

- Fruits alone (one to two hours).

- Starch (grains, root vegetables, beans, cereals, breads) go well with vegetables (three hours).

- Protein (nuts, seeds, beans, flesh) goes well with vegetables (four hours). *note:* Animal protein can take eight hours or longer.

- Protein and starch do not combine well. Examples: eggs and toast, peanut butter and bread (jelly too), nuts and grains.

- Protein and fruit do not combine well; neither do starch and fruit. Think overalls and a lacy bra. The overalls are like a slab of meat, the bra, a bowl of berries. Together they make a putrefaction disco!

- Though avocados are technically a fruit that's loaded with protein and good fats, they fall in the starch category. But these little gems (aka nature's butter) go with just about everything. Enjoy!

- Veggies are like Switzerland—totally neutral and go with everything. They are the glue that holds us together (two to three hours).

- Though fruit should really be eaten alone, you can make juices and smoothies with fruit and veggies.

HOT crazy*Sexy* TIP

Chewing thoroughly will help you absorb your food better and release waste with ease. In fact, some nutrition experts say you should drink your food and chew your water, which basically means that everything that goes down your throat should be pureed, because digestion starts with enzymes released in your saliva when you chew. So start grinding those purdy jaws! Sorry, fellow boozers, but another tip to remember is to try not to consume liquids while eating. They dilute the digestive juices. Remember to stop eating three hours before sleeping and not to stuff yourself. Leave room for joy, creativity, fun—and sex!

BEANS

You may be wondering why I put beans in the starch category in the combo basics sidebar. Technically, beans are both a starch and a protein. When you soak your beans overnight, you make them easier to digest. The same holds true for nuts and seeds. Soaking times vary. Usually the more dense the nut, the longer you'll need to soak it. You can easily find recommended soaking times online. For beans, add a 2-inch piece of kombu (seaweed) to the soaking water and those protein-packed fart generators will be even easier on your belly. Sprouting beans activates their life force, making them more like a nutritious veggie. Since beans are in both categories, you can combine them with starches (example: rice and beans). This goes for tofu and tempeh as well.

When in food-combining doubt, take a good digestive enzyme supplement, especially when consuming flesh. I take enzymes with each meal and have seen a drastic decline in the gas, bloating, and post-chow energy lag. (I'll talk more about these in chapter 9.)

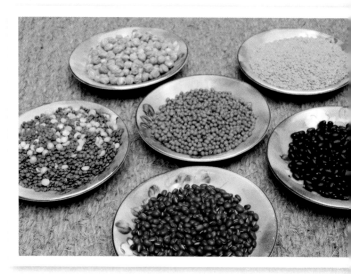

MORE ON BACTERIA

At this very moment, you're host to a mind-blowing microscopic menagerie of critters in your gut. Trillions of bacteria make up your intestinal flora, living and dying and doing jobs so important that you couldn't survive without them. There are so many, in fact, that they outnumber the cells of your actual body by ten to one. Among their vital roles: They produce specific hormones, enzymes, and vitamins (like K and certain Bs) that your body needs but wouldn't get otherwise, they break down fiber and gases, and they produce disease-fighting antibodies and help train the immune system. Clearly, these little dudes are our friends. But as we've already discussed, when our intestinal flora is imbalanced, we become more susceptible to a host of problems including digestive issues, asthma, allergies, infections, weight gain, hormonal imbalances, and many other issues in the tissues.

It's highly competitive in Bowel Town. In fact, you're host to a constant struggle for supremacy between good and bad, and your diet decides who wins. According to Marcelle Pick, OB/GYN NP and cofounder of womentowomen.com, "Intestinal microbes can die off by the millions with illness, stress, medication use, and poor diet, but what we eat is the most important factor in keeping the gut healthy. Good bacteria feast on fiber. The bad guys love refined sugar and animal fat."

You're like a weapons dealer who takes sides with every meal. Your intestinal climate affects virtually every aspect of your health. Whose side are you on?

> **Trillions of bacteria make up your intestinal flora, living and dying and doing jobs so important that you couldn't survive without them.**

BAKING BREAD IN YOUR BODY

For many pill-popping, boozing, sugar- and bagel-loving gals, yeast overgrowth, also called candida, is an issue. Candida comes in many different forms;

the little yeasties exist in small quantities as part of healthy gut flora. But when this nasty and opportunistic microorganism gets out of hand, it will take over any weak area of the body. Think Gremlins on crack! And guess what? Yeast makes its own poop, too. So not only are you dealing with your own waste, you're dealing with theirs, in the form of alcohol, formaldehyde, and other toxins.

How does yeast take over? You guessed it: overacidification of your inner landscape. In fact, it's next to impossible to rid yourself of a candida overgrowth if mercury is found in your system (usually from fish or dental fillings). Yeast have a major crush on mercury. They're like Edward and Bella from the *Twilight* series—inseparable! If you decide to have your amalgam fillings removed and replaced with nontoxic versions, make sure to find a holistic dentist with experience with this procedure. I did and have seen quite a difference.

Common symptoms of an intestinal yeast overgrowth include gas, bloating, mental fog, fatigue, weight gain, and headaches. Check yourself: White spots on the skin, nail and toe fungus, vaginal infections, or a coated tongue, may be signaling a demonic bakery on the inside! Once you have an overgrowth, it takes time and complete consistency to rebalance.

Vaginal yeast infections—otherwise known as baking bread or making cottage cheese in your bloomers—can be a sign of high blood sugar or diabetes. The yeast thrive on the extra sugar (so do the bacteria that cause bladder infections). Get a medical checkup, especially if you're overweight or menopausal.

Not to worry, the Crazy Sexy Diet plan is like voodoo for yeast. That's right, eating more alkaline foods is key. Yeast just love sugar and the acidity it causes, and that's exactly what they won't be getting. They don't get an opportunity to grow, because now you're eating very little sugar, no refined carbs, and loads of minerals, and you're focused on maintaining proper alkalinity and eliminating old, oxygen-sucking sludge.

If you suspect an intestinal yeast overgrowth, there are several natural remedies that can help. I use a combination of raw garlic (about one clove per day) and oregano oil capsules while avoiding all fruit, grains, breads, and carbs for a period of time. Candex and Candigone are good products that can be found in most health food stores. For more information, read *The Body Ecology Diet* by Donna Gates with Linda Schatz, a terrific book that can totally transform your terrain. Stick with her vegan suggestions if possible, and say bye-bye bugs, hello health!

IT'S IN the CRAPPER!

The beauty of the CSD is that after just a short while, you won't even think about being constipated (and all the negatives that go with it) or bloated. It just doesn't happen, and if it does, it's rare and you now know how to deal with it. Power to the pooper, baby! What's even more exciting for the whole digestive superhighway is the green elixir—juice. We're getting our juices flowing in the next chapter.

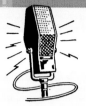

testimonial: Jessy F.

I started the CSD because I was indulging in waaaaay too many snacks, treats, and breads. I was addicted to sugar and bingeing late at night; as a result I was sluggish, depressed, and suffering from IBS. A normal day for me was visiting the bathroom at least twelve times. I had lived like this since I was twelve years old, and had enough.

I've been vegan since January 1, 2008—but giving up sugar, Diet Coke, and bread as I knew it (with gluten) was downright scary. At the end of week one I felt great and my IBS was nonexistent. I look forward to my morning juice 'n' smoothie, a giant salad for lunch, and mostly raw dinners. I've stayed gluten-free, mostly sugar-free, and no more sodas and junk. I feel too good to go back to the way I ate before. I do more yoga and the best part is I'm not in the bathroom twelve times a day. I feel happy, full of energy, and awesome!

CHAPTER 5 IN REVIEW

REMEMBER:

- You are what you eat and what you don't poop.
- Ingesting bad foods and toxins creates congestion in the digestion—and that's just the beginning of your problems.
- Enemas and colonics help take the trash out.
- Food combining is another great way to keep things moving.
- A balance in gut flora makes a healthy, happy you.

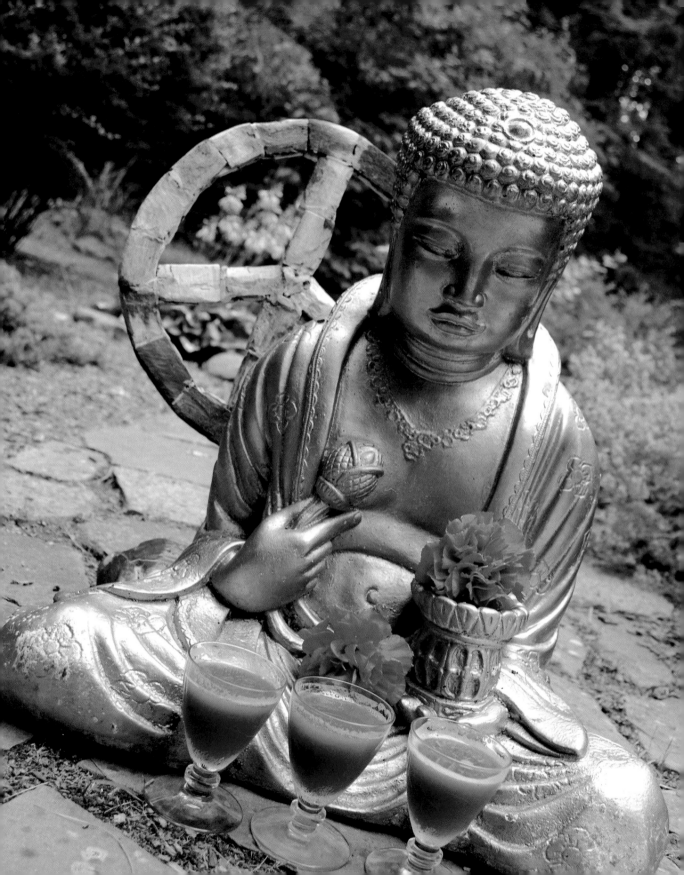

MAKE JUICE, NOT WAR

If you really want to get into the sparkle zone, you gotta get gaga for liquid nutrition! Organic green juice is like red lipstick; don't leave home without it. Juice is the muse and the medicine. Juice is also one of the best-kept beauty secrets around. Whether you're a Maybelline-wearing drugstore cowgirl or a Christian Dior debutante, you're wasting your money if you don't get with the Green Goddess. And it gets better, girls: Juicing helps to slow and even reverse the aging process. It reduces inflammation, cleanses the body, regulates the bowels, and can even help peel off extra pounds.

As my mentor, the 900-year-old Jedi Master Yoda, says, "May the Force be with you." Well, in this wet and juicy chapter you'll learn how to channel the Force through the power of juicing, blending smoothies, fasting, and hydration. By blessing your God pod with liquid love, you send a profound message to your cells: I got your back, and I adore you!

JUICING JEWELS

For some, the idea of drinking emerald-green liquid first thing in the morning is glorious. Cheers! To others, green juice, also known as "swamp in a glass," is totally barf-a-delic; you'd rather juice a bag of Cheetos or a fluffernutter sandwich than drink that shit. I've definitely been in your high heels. Drop the drama. It won't kill you. In fact, it will save you, so ease up, Grande Dame. Just because it's green doesn't mean it's gross—many veggies are actually quite sweet. The cleaner you get, the more your taste buds will change. Those little suckers literally come back to life. What once seemed nasty will become your deepest, most primal craving. Green blood rules!

Guzzling green goodness balances your pH and gives you a direct shot of vitamins, minerals, enzymes, protein, and oxygen. The trillions of cells in your glorious body are constantly being replaced—by the time seven years have passed, just about every cell in your body is new. Juicing helps you rebuild using the best raw materials on the planet. By removing the plant fiber during the juicing process, we instantly lighten the load on our digestion.

Within minutes of downing your green juice shot, your body receives a blast of optimum fuel that nourishes your cells and helps restore your immune system. I drink 16 to 32 ounces of fresh, organic green juice every day and wowza, is my body grateful. Think about how many cucumbers, kale leaves, and celery stalks it takes to make 16 to 32 ounces of juice—a lot! It would be nearly impossible to eat that much in one sitting, but with juice, you get the nutrients without stuffing yourself.

But wait, no fiber? Won't my blood sugar go wild? There's a common concern that juicing will cause your blood sugar to spike, since you're taking in sugar rapidly and without fiber to slow the process. My response is that with green juice the spike is minimal in comparison with fruit juice and juices that are heavy on carrot, beets, or apples. There will be a slight raise in blood sugar, of course, but nothing to worry about too much. Also, as you recall the GI rating of veggies is zero, so it really depends on what else you include.

By the way, it's best to drink your juice on an empty stomach. Mixing liquids with solids slows down the digestive process. It's better to have your juice and wait about thirty to forty-five minutes before eating solid food.

Cucumbers make a dazzling base for juicing. They're a terrific source of vitamin C and are highly alkalizing and cleansing. These water-filled wonders have a mildly sweet, kind flavor that's easy on the tummy. If you get nauseous or your belly is sensitive to stronger greens or veggies, beginning your juicing journey with a cukes-only cocktail is a nice way to ease in. Push one or two through your juicer and voilà—you've got a powerful healing elixir! Organic cucumbers can be juiced with the skins. The conventional kinds need to be peeled first, *por favor,* as they are covered with food-grade wax and pesticide residue.

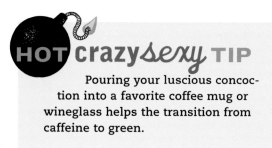

HOT crazysexy TIP

Pouring your luscious concoction into a favorite coffee mug or wineglass helps the transition from caffeine to green.

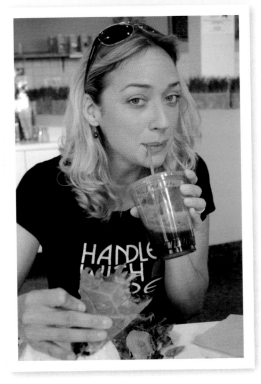

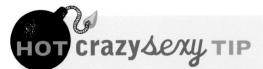

HOT crazy sexy TIP

You can whip up some ginger tea by grating the root and squeezing the juice (either through a cheesecloth or with your hand) into a cup of hot water.

When you're ready to kick it up a notch, add a few stalks of savory celery, a great source of minerals (especially potassium) and B vitamins. Please use only organic celery, as the conventional kind is loaded with icky sticky pesticides. (I'll discuss organic veggies in more detail in chapter 8.) Once you've come to love this classic combo, start adding big leafy greens and other veggies, one at a time. That way you'll go from a SAD slump to GLAD cartwheels without too much gastric grief. I love sweet-tasting miracle workers like romaine lettuce, pea sprouts, and broccoli stems. Build up to stronger-tasting, more medicinal plants like kale, chard, fennel, watercress, dandelion, cabbage, beet greens, cilantro, spinach, garlic, parsley, and ginger (but not all at once!).

A helpful word of warning about ginger, garlic, and parsley: A little goes a long way, warrior princess! These highly charged veggie shamans make magic, but have extremely strong flavors when juiced. A couple of tablespoons of freshly chopped parsley leaves, half a clove of garlic, or a piece of ginger half the size of your thumb is all you need at

first. More than that will blow your head off (just kidding—sorta).

For added sweetness, add carrot, beet, red or orange bell pepper, or low-glycemic fruit such as a small apple or pear to your recipes. Exact amounts vary depending on your serving size. A good rule of thumb is a 3:1 ratio: three veggies to one piece of fruit. Use this ratio when juicing carrots and beets as well, as they have a fair amount of sugar. (FYI: Beets may turn your poop a little reddish. Don't worry, there's no need to haul your ass to the emergency room.) Another popular juice gem is a little peeled lemon or other citrus, which cuts the bitterness of harsh greens for those aforementioned Grande Dames having a hard time.

So what about all the fiber that's left over in the pulp? Isn't it good for me? Yes, juicing does remove fiber, but it doesn't mean you won't get it elsewhere. If you're following my other recommendations, you are definitely consuming more than enough through all the whole or gluten-free grains, salads, steamed and sautéed veggies, beans, and other intestinal brooms.

Speaking of leftover pulp, it can feel wasteful to dump all those ground-up goodies into the garbage. But there are several things you can do to extract the most value from your veggies. First, try passing the pulp through the juicer a second time. Just remove the catch basket, dump the pulp into a bowl, grab it by the sloppy handful, and shove it back down the chute.

A $4 widemouthed canning funnel is a great way to make this process far less messy. Even with the best juicers, don't be surprised when a second pass squeezes that extra half a glass. That adds up to a lot of pennies over time, especially if you're buying organic. I don't bother with a third pass because at that point you're left with mostly dry fiber. Fresh pulp can also be used in various recipes, including soup stock, raw crackers, raw nut pâté, quick breads, and veggie patties. And finally, if you're able to compost, nothing makes sexier soil than veggie juice pulp—your garden will have an orgasm.

Here's a question I get asked a lot: Can't I just skip the whole juicing escapade, buy a bottle of the stuff, and call it a day? No, you can't, lazy bones. Prepackaged store-bought juices have little to no benefit—their nutrients are almost nil. Pasteurized juices may have a longer shelf life, but because they've been cooked at over 145 degrees they lack life force, aka enzymes. Remember, too, that many bottled juices are loaded with sugar, artificial colors, flavors, and preservatives. That's a recipe for an acid bath and a candida disco, if you ask me.

Whenever you start something new, it can be overwhelming. Let yourself be inspired by this juicy world of juicing. Channel your inner artist and get creative with your mixtures. Experiment with lots of combinations till you find the yummy groove that makes your taste buds sing like a bird. You can't make a mistake and you have nothing to lose—except weight, disease, and suffering.

A good rule of thumb is a 3:1 ratio: three veggies to one piece of fruit.

CHOOSE THE RIGHT JUICER

Choosing a juicer is like choosing a mate—it has to work with your lifestyle for the long haul. Lame juicers (and lovers) mean no foreplay, no blindfolds, and no juice.

There's a wide price range of juicers to choose from, but quality is sometimes the trade-off. The cheapest ones are often designed poorly, which means more juice ends up on you than in you. Their weak motors struggle with denser foods, like carrots, and don't yield much juice from leafy greens. At the other end of the spectrum are the pro machines. They can be overkill—as big and powerful as a truck, but costing more than a Gucci blouse! Personally, I'll take the blouse. Is there a happy medium? Yes—read on.

TOP JUICER BRANDS

There are lots of different juicer brands to choose from. Check out crazysexylife.com, discount juicers.com, bestjuicers.com, harvestessentials.com, and even amazon.com for thrifty buys.

MY TOP CHOICES ARE:

CENTRIFUGAL: Breville Ikon multispeed, Breville Juice Fountain Compact, Omega 4000

MASTICATING: Champion Juicer, Hurom Slow juicer

TWIN GEAR: Green Star Juice Extractor, Samson Ultra Juicer

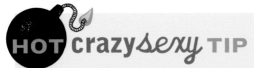
Bag it! If you can't afford another piece of equipment at this time, dig out that old blender from the back of the kitchen cabinet. Next stop: the hardware store. Pick up some paint strainer bags. They usually cost well under a dollar—a fraction of the cost for the juice-straining bags sold online and at some health food stores. Once you've blended, strain the juice through the fine-mesh bag into a bowl, squeezing it to get every drop of green gold out. Then get that chlorophyll in your sassy pants—drink the juice right away. Wash the bag out, use it a couple more times, and then compost it.

Consumer-quality juicers generally fall into three categories: centrifugal, masticating, and twin gear. What's the difference, and how do you choose? Here's the skinny:

Centrifugal juicers use a fast-spinning grater to shred the fruits and veggies. The juice then gets flung through a strainer and out the spout, while the pulp flies up and into a catch basket.

Masticating juicers use one slowly turning screw-shaped gear that chews up the veggies and squeezes the juice through a stainless-steel screen. This action gently tears open the cell membranes in order to release the nutrients.

Twin gear juicers are the crème de la crème. They work at even lower speeds, slowly squishing the fruits and veggies between two gears until the pulp is nearly dry and almost all the juice is squeezed out.

All three types have pros and cons. Centrifugal juicers are easy to use, quick to clean, and less expensive. Many of them have a wider mouth, which

means less prep time cutting and juicing veggies. However, the grating and spinning of centrifugal juicers causes the nutrients to oxidize quicker. Exposed to air, the enzymes start to break down and your juice loses some of its nutritional oomph. All juice should be consumed as quickly as possible, but this is especially true for those made in a centrifugal juicer. Consume them within fifteen to twenty minutes of juicing. If you can't drink it right away, don't wig out. Do what you can. Immediately pour your liquid sunshine in an airtight mason jar (fill to the top) and store it in your fridge for later.

Masticating juicers extract more juice. Because they operate at slower speeds than the whirling dervish centrifugal juicers, you get more nutrition (enzymes included), less foam, and a longer fridge life. If you need to, you can store your well-sealed juice for a day or so.

Twin-gear juicers give you the biggest bang for the buck. The juice lasts up to seventy-two hours (so they say). You can also use them to make scrumptious nut butters and even ice cream. Twins can also extract wheatgrass juice (as can some masticating juicers).

The downside is that both masticating and twin-gear models take longer to make juice and longer to clean up because they have a narrower mouth, move slower, and have more parts to scrub. They're also heavier and take up more counter space. And lastly, they're pricey. But they do make the best juice. Be nice, ask Santa, see what happens. Ultimately, the best juicer is the one you'll use! Juicers are not dust collectors, folks. They are active members of your family and they hate being shelved. Quite frankly, it hurts their feelings.

PASS THE GRASS

Wheatgrass juice is a powerful tonic for healing, as you learned in the preceding chapter. Those
magic mini-lawns are filled with liquid sunshine,
crammed with chlorophyll. According to *The Wheatgrass Book* by Ann Wigmore (the queen mum of
chlorophyll), wheatgrass juice "Increases red blood-
cell count and lowers blood pressure. It cleanses the
blood, organs and gastrointestinal tract of debris.
Wheatgrass also stimulates metabolism. The juice's
abundance of alkaline minerals helps reduce overacidity in the blood. It can be used to relieve many
internal pains, and has been used successfully to
treat peptic ulcers, ulcerative colitis, constipation,
diarrhea, and other complaints of the gastrointestinal tract. The enzymes and amino acids found in
wheatgrass can protect us from carcinogens like
no other food or medicine. It strengthens our cells,
detoxifies the liver and bloodstream, and neutralizes
environmental pollutants."

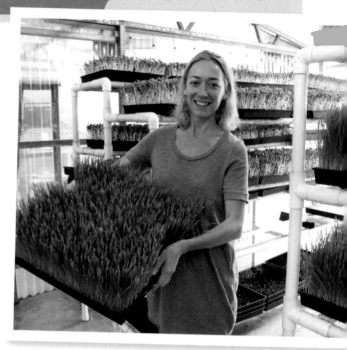

For fresh wheatgrass, check your local health
food store, or grow your own. You can buy inexpensive, easy-to-use wheatgrass growing kits from
many online sources. Some even come with the soil.
Visit my pal Michael Bergonzi's (the wheatgrass
king) Web site to learn everything you ever wanted
to know about this magical grass: wheatgrassgreen
house.com.

He's the best grower in the country and will
teach you a ton about sprouting, too. In the age of
online shopping, you can get trays of fresh wheatgrass shipped right to your door. To enjoy DIY
wheatgrass juice at home, you'll need a twin-gear
juicer or a not-so-fancy hand-crank model. That's
what I use—it's a little plastic job that I got for
$28—great for travel and easy to clean. Go to
healthyjuicer.com for more deets.

BLEND, BABY, BLEND

Another great way to get liquid nutrition is to blend your fruits and veggies into delicious green smoothies. They're easy to make, take little prep and cleanup time, and require only one piece of kitchen equipment—a blender! The difference between a juice and a smoothie is that a smoothie leaves no pulp behind—it contains all the fantastic fiber of the ingredients. The tough cellulose structure of the produce is broken into tiny pieces that are easy for your body to digest and assimilate.

Think of it as a pre-chewed blast of optimum nutrition. Smoothies balance pH and blood sugar while the fiber assists in sponging up toxins. You can load them up with good fats, quality vegan protein powders (see supplement chapter), and ground flax, chia, or hemp seeds. Smoothies are more filling and provide more energy. On days when I want rich and creamy emotional comfort, I blend, baby, blend!

There are a million ways to make a smoothie and even more recipes online. I call my enlightened fave "the Green Guru." It's like wisdom in a glass! The guru's ingredients are really simple: avocado, coconut water (or purified water), cucumber, romaine, pear or banana, a dash of stevia (or agave), a wee bit of cinnamon or cacao, and 1 to 2 ounces of E3Live (see chapter 9 for more on this supplement).

When building your smoothies, it's best to use the same 3:1 (veggie to fruit) ratio as described for juice. Berries are a good low-glycemic choice in the summer (put 'em in the freezer for added pizzazz). Sweet pea or sunflower sprouts are electric—they're loaded with oxygen and protein. Other lovely leafy options include spinach, kale, and red lettuce.

BLENDER BARGAINS

Now that you've got the blending scoop, do you have the right tools? Like most people, I had an old hand-me-down blender from my mom's disco daiquiri days. You know the one—cracked pitcher, missing buttons, and a motor with the power of a nose hair trimmer. I didn't know what I was missing until I got serious about green smoothies. I now use a Vita-Mix, the Cadillac of blenders. This sucker could pulverize a cowboy boot! I use it to make the creamiest smoothies, soups, puddings, dressings, sauces, and occasional (killer!) margarita. The only drawback is the price: anywhere from $340 to over $600, depending on the model. But it'll be the last blender you ever buy! Snag one when you get a little financial breathing room.

The Blendtec is another powerful high-end brand. They're slightly less expensive, starting at around $230 and going up to $600. Among smoothie aficionados there are those in the Vita-Mix camp and others firmly planted in the Blendtec camp—it's up to you to decide. Always do research, read consumer reviews, and Internet- and comparison-shop for the best deals.

As for moderately priced blenders, Breville has three models ranging from $150 to $300. Waring's MBB518 Pro is less than $200 and gets user kudos for strength and durability. KitchenAid's five-speed, 56-ounce blender is less than $100 and earns high marks. And at around $65, the Oster Classic Beehive is a stylin' bargain.

JUICING VERSUS BLENDING

Is juicing better than blending? I recommend including both in your weekly repertoire. Both are terrific, but juice gives you instant energy while smoothies take a bit longer to assimilate and require more work from your body. Personally, I juice more than I blend. In an average week I'll juice four to five days and enjoy smoothies for the remainder. Juice makes me feel lighter and more hydrated first thing in the morning. Breakfast literally means "to break a fast" and I prefer to do that with juice. It allows my body a longer process of cleansing and repair.

But I don't want to give green smoothies a bad rap. They are definitely more filling and stick with you longer, plus they take less time to make. They're also an easier sell to skeptics. In 2009 I went to New Orleans to care for displaced female survivors of Hurricane Katrina with my friends from the Urban Zen Foundation. We spent three days in the Superdome as part of Eve Ensler's ten-year V-day anniversary. The stadium was transformed into SUPERLOVE—a place to heal, celebrate, and activate through yoga, massage, healing circles, makeovers, and more.

I made smoothies—anywhere between 5,000 and 7,000 cups of liquid love! The SUPERLOVE recipe was really simple: cucumber, watermelon, a sprig of mint, a dash of agave sweetener, and ice. Normally, I wouldn't add sweetener to a recipe like this, but the fabulous gals of the Big Easy were used to sugar and spice and everything not so nice. As a result, many of them had serious health issues.

My goal was to teach the women that real fruits and veggies can be delicious. If added sweetener could help me do it, amen! In the end I was surprised at the number of ladies who came back for seconds and thirds. I highly doubt I would have nabbed so many skeptics with a dark green glass of juice. The moral of this story is that luscious smoothies can be the sneaky little helper you need to get your friends and family to embrace healthy libations.

The bottom line: Do what works best for your majestic self (and your schedule). Including liquid nutrition, in whatever form, will change your life. Juice, blend, sip, somersault. Got it?

FASTING

Fasting is nature's surgical table. It's also a ticket to the divine. Fasting affects you on every level—physical, mental, emotional, and spiritual. This ancient practice has a long history in culture and religion. But like many time-honored wisdoms that have been bleached from our society, fasting gets a bad rap these days. It's considered either a fad, new agey, or dangerous. But we can look to the animal kingdom to learn the truth about the "dangers" of fasting.

When my super-pooch Lola gets a bellyache from sneaking rotten treats from the garbage or dining on deer turd, she doesn't call up the vet or head to the drugstore. She fasts by drinking water and chewing grass and is feeling better posthaste. Quite frankly, I'd rather take a page from her healing manual than get sucked into the medical system of endless pills, bills, and insurance bullshit.

Fasting should never equal starvation, deprivation, or restriction. Fasting is simply resting from solid food. You'll still be receiving an enormous amount of nutrition (and oxygen!) in liquid form. Fasting gives your body a break from spending the enormous amounts of energy required to break down food—especially the high quantities of junk in the Standard American Diet—and allows you to redirect that energy toward healing and detoxification. While fasting, you release toxins stored in your colon, liver, lungs, bladder, sinuses, skin, and kidneys, allowing your body to function better.

On my 21-Day Plan (see chapter 10), I recommend fasting one day per week. I base my protocol on personal experience and what I learned during my health educator training at the Hippocrates Health Institute. In his book *Living Foods for Optimum Health,* Dr. Brian Clement, director at Hippocrates, says, "Fast one day every week, consuming only freshly squeezed green drinks, vegetable juices, purified water, herbal teas. These fasting days will allow any potential long-term toxins to be released before they can cause serious damage. It's like changing the oil in your car before your engine fails."

Do you need to fast in order to cleanse your body? No, at least not at first. Depending on your current diet, abstaining from meat, dairy, processed sugars, and starches while adding alkaline food and drink may be all you need to help eliminate the garbage in your system. Once you've leaned into a better diet, then you can kick it up a notch with a fast. If you go from 0 to 60 too quickly, you may find the experience overly intense (more on detox symptoms in a jiffy). Fasts are not a quick fix or a magic bullet. You know how I feel about those—they don't work! You'll fall flat on your face and gain the weight or

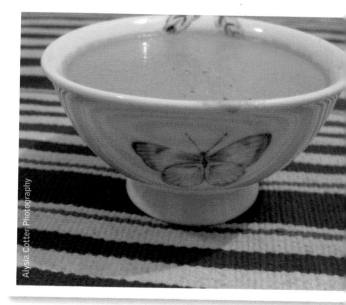

Alysia Cotter Photography

dis-ease back. Are we on the same page? Fasting only works in conjunction with a better overall diet that's consumed on a consistent basis.

Fasting only works in conjunction with a better overall diet that's consumed on a consistent basis.

A DAY IN THE LIFE OF A HEALTHY FAST

Hydrate, nourish, hydrate! This is the mantra for a healthy fast. Drink lots of green nourishment, purified water with lemon and herbal teas. When I fast, I drink about 64 to 92 ounces of fresh, organic green juice—about 16 ounces at each sitting. This may be too much for you. If your fast includes smoothies, you probably won't need as many ounces since smoothies are bulkier than juices. Just make sure you get enough and that you're not too hungry. A little pang is fine, but no meltdowns! If your belly gurgles, drink more water or have a cup of herbal tea. After twenty-four hours, ease out of the fast with a green smoothie or a blended raw soup made with veggies, herbs, and spices.

A teaspoon per serving of good fat—such as hemp, flax, or olive oil—makes soups rich and creamy. If you prefer, you can use half an avocado instead of oil. Some people find raw soups to be more palatable if they're slightly chilled (see the recipes in chapter 10 for ideas and inspiration). If you prefer warm soups, blend them in your Vita-Mix until the veggies start to heat up. This rapid stirring raises the temperature a bit without losing many nutrients. You can also warm your soup slightly on the stove. Use your finger as a thermometer. If the soup's too hot for your digit, it's too hot for you (and the enzymes, vitamins, minerals, etc.)!

The ingredients used in my simple sexy juice fast can vary; you don't need to stick to them exactly. Just as in life, variety is the spice that makes us sing. So switch your recipes around to avoid mind-bending boredom, screaming at public utility workers, or grand theft auto! Drink as much as you like and remember to not only change the menu to suit your palate, but rotate your veggies to make sure you're getting all your vitamins and minerals.

A SIMPLE *sexy* ONE-DAY JUICE FAST

7 A.M.: 8 ounces water with lemon and a pinch of cayenne. This cleanses your liver and stimulates circulation. If you like, sip your favorite herbal tea throughout the day.

8–9 A.M.: 16 to 20 ounces of green juice: cucumber, celery, broccoli stems, kale, romaine, one pear, ½-inch piece of gingerroot.

11 A.M.: Midmorning pick-me-up: 16 to 20 ounces of green juice.

1 P.M.: Lunch. You guessed it—16 to 20 ounces green juice.

4 P.M.: Afternoon delight. Oh my, what could it be? 16 to 20 ounces green juice. If possible, also suck back a 2- to 4-ounce shot of wheatgrass!

6–7 P.M.: For dinner, you can continue with just juice, a smoothie, or blended raw soup. If you're feeling too uncomfortable or prefer to ease out of your fast with solid food, have a light salad or some gently steamed veggies with a little olive oil and sea salt or a bowl of miso soup with well-chopped greens and scallions.

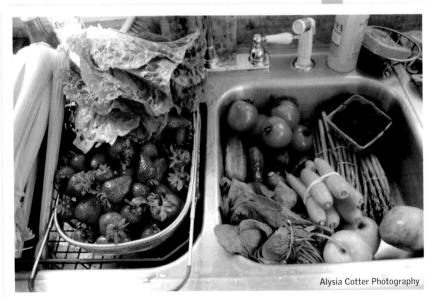

Alysia Cotter Photography

Though you will be drinking lots of green nutrition, don't be surprised if you hit a few icy patches. The more toxins you've accumulated, the more you'll have to eliminate. Detox symptoms occur because toxins are leaving the cells and tissues faster than the body can eliminate them, and for many that can spell discomfort and a lot of toilet time. This is natural, but if it gets too intense you can easily dial it down. Folks living on McDonald's, Dunkin's, and Doritos might have a lot of discomfort as the demons exorcise.

In all honesty a one-day fast shouldn't cause too much drama. Uncomfortable symptoms are a bigger problem on longer fasts. That said, expect some mucus, skin eruptions, headaches, stinky gas, a thick white coating on the tongue, and fatigue. You may even experience some nausea. Once you get over the healing hump, you will feel much better. When symptoms arise, remember to drink lots of water to help flush you out.

Here's something else to remember: Poisons drain your energy. When you release them, you also release their patterns—including the mental, emotional, and spiritual chaos they cause. Emotional swings are common during juice cleansing—yes, even within a twenty-four-hour period. As with the physical symptoms, grab a box of tissues and ride them out.

It's also a good idea to follow a fast with an enema (or a colonic) to keep the pipeline clear, allowing for better evacuation going forward. For a good sweat, sit your cute butt in the sauna, too! If you think fasting is too extreme for you, then honor that feeling. But I ask you to pause for a moment and consider what many of us deem normal—gallstones and gallbladder removal, blood pressure medicine, insulin pumps, debilitating arthritis,

HOT crazysexy TIP

An important tip for long-term fasters: Failure to maintain your electrolytes can be dangerous. However, the solution is simple: Add a pinch of sea salt to your juice, or make sole and drink the salt water.

steroids, and other medical miseries. A plant-based diet and some periodic housekeeping seem pretty easy to me!

LONGER FASTS

Some folks do longer fasts, but keep in mind that longer is not always better. Long-term fasting must also be accompanied by regular colonics. My longest green drink fast was twenty-one days. It was a detox dump-a-thon! My liver deep-sixed garbage, my lymph yacked, and my butt exorcised the demon. As my colon hydrotherapist said, "Here come the mummies!" But it was also a physical and emotional roller coaster.

My energy level went up, down, and back up again. Ultimately there were definite pluses and it served me well, but I do not recommend a long-term fast for most people, especially without expert supervision. Particularly because you really have to be careful about electrolyte imbalance and how you come off the fast. I've seen a few fasting enthusiasts replace one addiction for another. This isn't a marathon and there's no such thing as ultimate purity. In fact, let's not forget that stressing about perfection is as bad as booze, cigs, animal toes, and white crap.

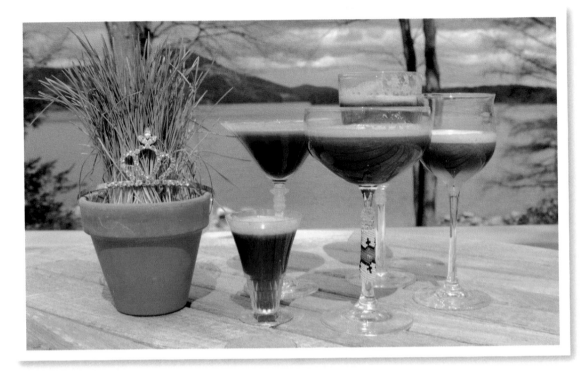

Some people should avoid fasting. If your current health is too weak or if you have an eating disorder, are underweight, or are being treated for a chronic disease such as cancer, if you have heart problems or are pregnant or lactating, fasting of any kind is not recommended. Also, children should never fast. Be realistic and honest. If you have any concerns, check with your doctor. Water fasts are not recommended. Water fasting will dump far too many stored poisons into our bloodstream at a rate that most of us simply cannot tolerate. The same goes for those popular water, maple syrup, cayenne, and vinegar fasts—that ain't nutrition.

WATER

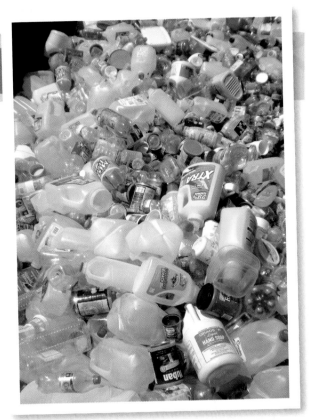

Drinking purified water is like giving your insides a bath, a good rinse, a happy shower. Refreshing! Besides, water is the best drink to quench your thirst—if you can get off the diet pop kick and replace it with water, you've accomplished a great deed. Our bodies are made up of over 70 percent water. Your brain is roughly 80 percent water. Remember, you're electric—when your cells don't have enough fluid, they lose their conductivity. Water helps nutrients flow into our cells and acid wastes flow out. Water is the main component of blood and lymph. It regulates body temperature. Water is absolutely essential to good health. Because we lose nearly 3 quarts a day through respiration, sweat, and urine, it's important to replenish daily.

Ideally, we should be consuming half our body weight in ounces of pure water each day. For example, a 140-pound person should drink 70 ounces (about nine 8-ounce glasses) throughout the day. It may seem like a lot, and certainly when you're juicing on a regular basis, drinking herbal teas, and eating lots of raw veggies, you don't need as much. To keep up with the demands of your inner ocean, it's best to pace yourself and sip throughout the day without waiting to feel thirsty. By the time you feel the sensation of thirst, you're already dehydrated. And hunger is often just a sign of thirst.

Oh, and guess what? Coffee is not water. Neither is black tea, soda, bottled juice, "vitamin water," or bullshit Red Bulls. These beverages actually pull water (and minerals) from your body. Don't have any illusions that you're quenching your thirst when you drink them.

Can you overdo it? Yes. If you act like a frat boy in a hazing ritual and chug an insane amount of water all at once, you can develop what's called water intoxication, also known as hyponatremia. It's extremely rare, with most cases occurring to overheated athletes. The point is, don't go crazy—just stay hydrated with moderate amounts of water at regular intervals.

BOTTLED WATER: JUST SAY NO

Although it's oh-so-convenient to buy bottled water, it's also a catastrophic waste on so many levels. Untold millions of plastic bottles clog our bloated landfills every year, and since space is extremely limited, we end up shipping our mountains of garbage to developing countries or simply dumping it far out to sea. Pound for pound, plastic bottles are one of the most ubiquitous forms of trash that pollute our oceans, rivers, roadways, and parks. Plastic bottles can last hundreds or even thousands of years. In turn, marine life and birds mistake plastic litter for food and end up choking and dying in droves.

If I haven't already gotten your attention, this might: That fancy $3 bottle of water is often nothing more than tap water. In fact, according to Food and Water Watch (foodandwaterwatch.org), tap water is actually better overall than most bottled water. The bottled water industry is subject to minimal regulation and oversight, and most bottling plants go uninspected for years on end. While the labels show serene and reassuring images of mountain glaciers and tropical waterfalls, you actually might just be guzzling from a big-city spigot or a hole drilled down the road from God-knows-what Superfund site.

Popular brands may contain the same toxic chemicals, pesticides, and pathogens that occur in tap water. And because the bottles aren't always sterilized before filling, that supposedly "clean" product could have nasty fungi and bacteria growing in it. Hey, did I mention that most bottled waters are acidic? It's true—many of the most popular brands test at a pH of around 5 or 6. Ultimately, you're spending up to 1,000 times more per gallon for bottled water than tap water.

Of course, if you're in a pinch it's best to stay hydrated by buying a bottle than to go without. But if you can make a modest investment in a water filter and a reusable stainless-steel bottle, like a Kleen Kanteen, then do yourself and the planet a favor and buy them. Stay away from the reusable hard plastic bottles. They contain dangerous chemicals known as BPAs, which can wreak havoc on our hormones. (Many other products contain BPAs, including baby bottles and food containers. Federal and state laws are beginning to restrict their use, but for now, it's best to stay vigilant. These plastics

FILTERED WATER TIPS

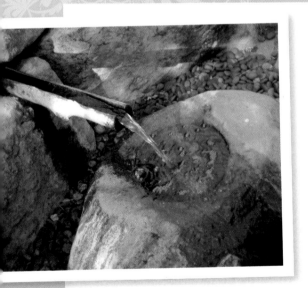

- Change filters periodically according to manufacturer's recommendations. A dirty filter not only doesn't work but can actually add impurities to your water. Mold likes carbon filters.

- Filtered water doesn't keep—refrigerate or use it soon after filtration. The nasty critters will grow back quicker than usual now that the chlorine has been removed.

- Fill ice cube trays with filtered water. Your cocktails (virgin or slut) will taste sooo much better.

- Rinse your fruits and veggies, and soak your nuts and seeds in filtered water.

- If you're in the middle of cancer treatments like chemo and radiation, you may want to use food-grade hydrogen peroxide (FGHP) to soak and clean your veggies.

FILTRATION METHODS

Almost all home water filtration systems use one of these two types of filters:

- **Activated carbon filters.** These work by passing water through tiny grains of charcoal, which attract and remove particulates. This system is effective on chlorine and most organic matter, but misses certain tiny chemical compounds, fluoride, and most metals.

- **Reverse osmosis (RO) filters.** These force water through a membrane that has extremely small holes—about one millionth the width of a human hair. This removes almost every dissolved solid, including many toxic chemicals. It's a slow process and wastes a lot, since only about 10 percent of the water entering the system makes it through.

can usually be identified by RECYCLE #7 printed on the bottom.)

PURE WATER AT HOME

Compared to many poor countries in the world, the tap water in the United States is definitely better, but don't think it's completely safe. According to a 2009 *New York Times* study, more than 20 percent of municipal water treatment systems violated key provisions of the Safe Drinking Water Act in the previous five years, exposing tens of millions of people to unsafe water. Keep in mind that this act only regulates 91 out of more than 60,000 chemicals in use in the United States.

A typical glass of tap water might contain a rogue's list of frightening things that shouldn't be there: heavy metals, industrial solvents, pesticides, rocket fuel, and even pharmaceuticals your neighbors peed down their drains in the past. The chlorine that is put in the water to kill germs is itself controversial, because it also kills your intestinal flora. For the millions of homes relying on well water, unfortunately the story isn't much different (except for the chlorine).

What to do? Install a water filter. While no filter guarantees absolutely purity, they can be a great improvement. Different types of filters remove or reduce different types of impurities. To figure out what you need, learn about your water first. Start by requesting your community's annual water-quality report, available from the utility or from your local health department. You should also test the water from your tap, since it may have picked up junk on its journey to your sink. Your local health department or an independent lab can do it for free or for a small fee.

Next, you'll want to consider which water you want to filter. Drinking only? Or cooking, bathing, and laundry as well? For most households, I recommend using filtered water at least for drinking and cooking. But keep in mind that your skin is your body's largest organ and you absorb many substances through it, so if you can filter your bathing water as well, brava! For maximum filtration, a whole-house system can be installed. These usually connect to the main pipe shortly after it enters the house and can be hidden out of sight in a basement or closet. For kitchen use only, there are smaller, under-sink models.

Filtration systems range in price from about $60 on up to $400 or more, and should be installed by a plumber—or that sexy somebody who's handy with tools. Finally, the simplest and cheapest way to treat drinking water is to buy a pitcher that contains a filter. Wellness Carafe, Brita, and Pur are three popular brands.

There is some debate about whether it's better to drink water that contains minerals or water that has been purified and the minerals removed. Trace amounts of essential calcium, magnesium, and sodium have been flowing in our mountain streams and nourishing us forever. So assuming you can still find clean, natural water, there's nothing wrong with it. But compared with your food, drinking water delivers only a tiny fraction of these important minerals. It's no big deal if you drink purified water, so long as you're also eating a healthy diet. Reverse osmosis and distillation are two common filtration methods that remove minerals. They can be remineralized with a pinch of quality sea salt.

A word of caution about distilled water: It's not as pure as commonly believed. In fact, any chemicals with a boiling point below water are not removed. This includes chlorine and many insecticides and herbicides.

IONIZED WATER

Some filter systems can also ionize the water—that is, use electrolysis to break the water into acid and alkaline portions. There are household uses for both. Acid water is good for washing veggies, as well as skin, hair, and brushing teeth, while alkaline water is good for juicing, cooking, and drinking. In the body alkaline water is said to help eliminate acid waste, balance pH, and act as an antioxidant by mopping up free radicals. Countertop and under-sink ionizing devices are widely available online. These units are fairly expensive ($1,000 to $3,000), but keep in mind they also contain carbon filters, so in a sense you're getting two filters for the price.

One last thought. If you don't filter your water, your body will—and your liver and kidneys will be very unhappy about it. Don't make them put in overtime. They need beauty sleep just like you, my lovely.

DRINKING BUDDIES

I'm a juicehead all right; I love my Green Goddess morning, noon, and night. I love to hydrate with clean, healing water. Let's be drinking buddies and (faux) egg each other on. You always drink more when you do it with a friend. How about enlisting a few other like-minded ladies (or gents) to swap recipes, check in to make sure you've met your daily goal, or just to toast to the new yous!

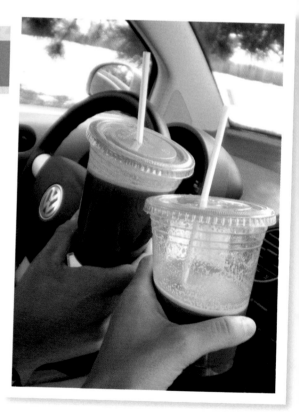

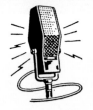

testimonial: Ryan R.

The Crazy Sexy Diet launched me into a fantastic journey. I had been struggling with a variety of issues that evolved during my radiation treatments last summer. The diet appealed to me because I was frustrated with not feeling like myself (a strong, nutritionally balanced, confident, vegetarian mother of four, wife, and science teacher). One major issue that I have suffered is with my voice. It has been hoarse or absent since I started radiation last June.

The daily juice and mostly raw diet has vastly improved the quality and strength of my voice. I am convinced that hydration is a major part of my voice issue. My radiologist insists that my voice issues can't be related to my treatments; however, in addition to laryngitis/severe hoarseness, I was incredibly thirsty from day one of radiation and tamoxifen. No amount of water intake quenched my thirst. The radiation ended in early August and I quit taking the tamoxifen in November.

Although I had been a vegetarian and had juiced vegetables regularly over the last thirty-plus years, I had never considered making green juice. Today, thanks to CSD, green juice is a major component of my daily diet. Cucumber is the base of my daily green breakfast cocktail. My dehydration issues are finally resolved! I am hopeful that with speech therapy my voice will recover. My diet is evolving toward vegan and I feel very well. I no longer fear the return of the cancer. I am confident that my improving diet will help me maintain my health.

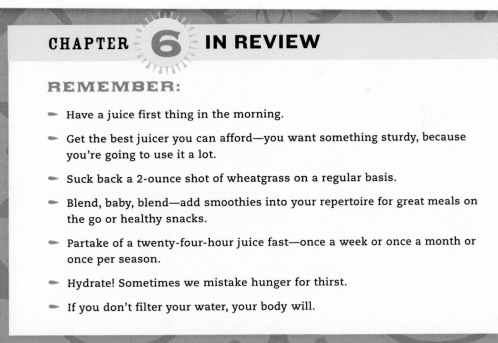

CHAPTER 6 IN REVIEW

REMEMBER:

- Have a juice first thing in the morning.

- Get the best juicer you can afford—you want something sturdy, because you're going to use it a lot.

- Suck back a 2-ounce shot of wheatgrass on a regular basis.

- Blend, baby, blend—add smoothies into your repertoire for great meals on the go or healthy snacks.

- Partake of a twenty-four-hour juice fast—once a week or once a month or once per season.

- Hydrate! Sometimes we mistake hunger for thirst.

- If you don't filter your water, your body will.

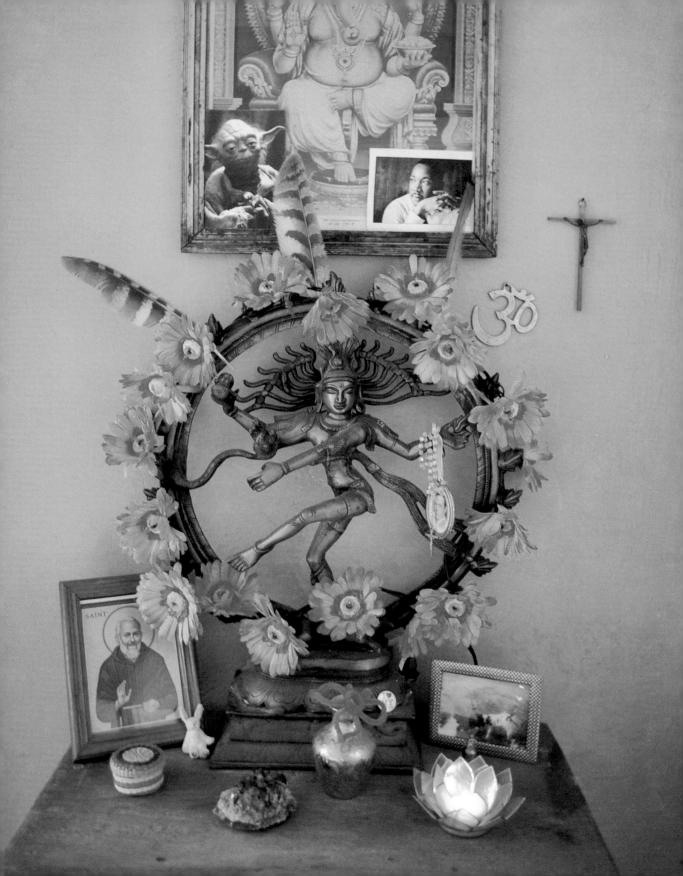

GOD POD GLOW

Self-care (including cleansing and detoxing) extends beyond the food in your fridge. A Crazy Sexy life includes reflection, booty shake, natural beauty products, rest, and relaxation. But you knew that, right? And yet it's so easy to overcommit or mismanage your time. Like most multitasking gals, you've probably broken many promises to yourself. You've written "Eat right and exercise more" resolutions for decades. As life spins out of control, you break those resolutions—often after just a few days of trying them. This all-too-common pattern sets the stage for a bigger problem.

The dilemma with continually falling on and off the self-care wagon isn't that you missed out on sweating, healthy food, soul pampering, and prayer, it's that you eventually lose trust in your own word. That's 911 bad. Losing trust leads to losing belief in your self-worth. Ouch! What's next? "Why bother? I never follow through," "I'll always be fat, sick, and unhappy," "I'm not good enough or smart enough," "It runs in my family, there's nothing I can do." Do you see the powerless position these words put you in? Enter the language police.

As hard as it might be, I want you to backtalk your inner nag and get on the wagon again. She doesn't deserve the last word. Your words (or hers!) create your reality. They affirm all things good or all things negative. This isn't just some

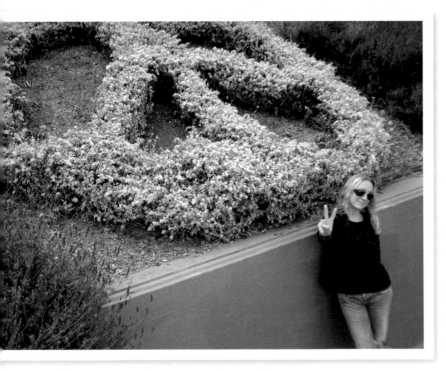

food, imagination time, and adventures into the wild. If playground bullies hurt her feelings, you'd hug her tears away and give her perspective. When tantrums or meltdowns turned her into a poltergeist, you'd demand a loving time-out in the naughty chair.

From this day forward I want you to extend the same compassion to your adult self. As Terri Cole, an awesome therapist, life coach, and my best pal, says, "If not you, then who? If not now, then when?" The next time your inner nag has something bad to say, stop and think about that kid. Then rewrite your script accordingly. You're worth it, angel wing. The world needs you to stand in your holy shazzam glory! Polish your inner and outer shine to a brilliant luster by committing to a comprehensive self-care regime.

new agey "Secret" shit; it's the key to creating harmony in your life. So as you approach this new anti-inflammatory diet and lifestyle, will you choose half-empty thinking or half-full? Here's a hint: Choose half full! Rebuild trust by showering yourself with kindness and care. Make space for the new you by cherishing your time and using it wisely. The world won't explode if you ease up, let go, and chillax. Stress sucks. It eats you alive. And if you're a perfectionistic control freak, I'm especially talking to you. Take things off your plate, dear one. Create new habits and new routines that support your highest good.

Here's a helpful exercise: Picture yourself when you were five. In fact, dig out a photo of little you at that time and tape it to your mirror. How would you treat her, love her, feed her? How would you nurture her if you were the mother of little you? I bet you would protect her fiercely while giving her space to spread her itty-bitty wings. She'd get naps, healthy

Like most multitasking gals, you've probably broken many promises to yourself.

Meditation
BOOT CAMP

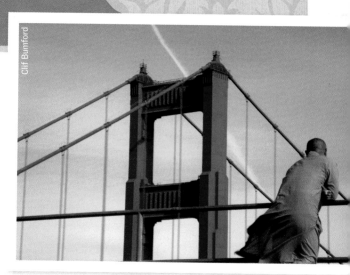
Clif Bumford

Meditation is a prerequisite for Crazy Sexy success. When your mind is strong and centered, cravings and emotional discomfort won't have the same sabotaging effect. Therefore, it stands to reason that a positive way to start your day looks something like this: pee, brush your teeth, and sit your ass on a meditation pillow! Wait, no coffee, news, or *New York Times*? Nope.

Our minds are the most open first thing in the morning. How we start our day sets us up for success or failure. As my friend Marianne Williamson says, "Do not be mystified about why you are depressed by noon when you start your day with the angst and despair in the world, especially if you add caffeine."

I recently gave a wellness lecture at Harvard University. Toward the end of my speech, I taught the students a simple meditation technique and encouraged them to join me for five minutes of silence. When the time was up, I asked the bright-minded kids how it felt. One of the young men made the following observation: "I hated it! Half-way through it felt like torture." Hold up, halfway through was at minute 2.5! "What if I told you that meditation could teach you how to better concentrate and focus, which would ultimately enhance your performance at school?" I asked. That got their attention! As you can imagine, Harvard is an extremely competitive joint where the vast majority of the students experience major burnout. What good is the expensive knowledge if you're too fried to use it? That day we began to strategize a curriculum for what I called the Inner Harvard. Naturally, meditation was at the top of the list. When you understand your mind you can harness its power

to achieve more than you imagined possible. The space between the noise is where God/dess lives. There are many answers there. Don't shy away from visiting.

Like the young Harvard student, the thought of meditating may overwhelm you. Some imagine excruciating boredom. Others are afraid of what they might feel if they took the time to pay attention. I can totally relate. In the past, wild maniac squatters frequently took up residence between my ears, under my blond hair. When I first started meditating I thought I would Helter Skelter snap.

Since then I've lived in monasteries, made pilgrimages to zendos, ashrams, sweat lodges, churches, mosques, and retreats. The silence within those walls reminded me that beneath my static lay an encyclopedia of healing guidance. Calm . . . can you picture it? What a nice place to take a day trip! It's free, and the view is spectacular. Start (and end) your day with five minutes, graduate to ten, work up to twenty, and so on. Meditation quiets the din and introduces you to yourself. "Hi me, I'm me, nice to meet you!"

THE BUSY PERSON'S
GUIDE TO . . . STOPPING

Before you jump in, here are a few suggestions that may prevent complete lunacy. Create a sacred space just for you. It doesn't have to be elaborate. We're not talking Taj Mahal here. My space consists of a little altar with pictures I love, candles, posies (altars like offerings), angel cards, and other spiritual tchotchkes. Christmas lights help, too. I like to meditate, pray, rant, and journal while sitting on a pillow in front of my altar. As soon as my butt hits the cushion, it's excavation time. If a pillow doesn't work for you, try a comfortable seat or a back jack chair (a floor chair that has fantastic back support). Buy a kitchen timer or a meditation chime. Set the timer for an appropriate number of minutes—ten to fifteen to start. Close your eyes and take a deep and cleansing breath in through your nose and out through your mouth. Let your breath settle into a normal rhythm and then begin to count to ten. Inhale one—exhale; inhale two—exhale; and so on. If that's too slow for you then inhale one—exhale two—inhale three—exhale four, etc. If your mind drifts and you imagine yourself buying shoes or guns, gently bring it back and start counting again. Your mind is like a muscle: The more consistent you are, the stronger you get.

Each time you return to the breath, you break an old pattern (distraction) and create a new mental habit (focus). Direct your mind where you want it to travel instead of always going for the ride. You can also use a mantra if this is easier for you. For example, inhale "let," exhale "go," or inhale "may all beings everywhere," exhale "be happy and free." When the timer beeps, you're done. You did it! Now do it again later and again tomorrow. Got it?

One last note: There is no "right" way to tune in. If a guided meditation or visualization works better for you, fantastic! There are countless CDs available. Chanting, Kirtan, and dance are other great tools. Check out my dear mentor and spiritual sister Gabrielle Roth's 5 Rhythms method, also known as "Sweat Your Prayers." Gabrielle's deeply healing movement meditation draws from shamanism, eastern philosophy, and psychology. At the core of the practice is the belief that everything is energy that moves in waves, patterns, and rhythms, which releases the heart and mind in order to connect to the soul. Amen! For more information, check out www.gabrielleroth.com.

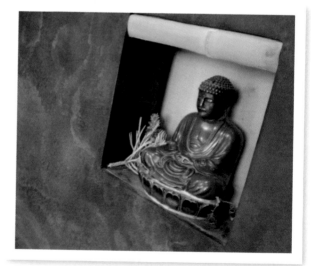

MORNING SADHANA

with Sharon Gannon

The Sanskrit word sadhana means to engage in conscious spiritual practice—doing something that brings you closer to the divine, closer to Self-realization, closer to enlightenment, closer to the truth of who you are and who the others in your life really are, closer to being a kinder person. For something to be *sadhana,* it must be practiced every day; it must become part of your life.

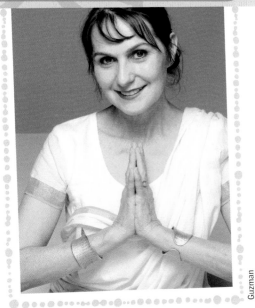

Guzman

My own morning *sadhana* begins very simply with a prayer and a promise: On awakening I stay in bed for a few minutes and remember to be thankful to God, saying silently: "Make me an instrument for Thy Will; not mine but Thine be done; free me from anger, jealousy, and fear; fill my heart with joy and compassion." I then silently recite the Sanskrit prayer *Lokah Samastah Sukino Bhavantu,* and follow with the English version: "May all beings everywhere be happy and free, and may the thoughts, words, and actions of my own life today contribute in some way to that happiness and to that freedom for all." In this way I have a precious opportunity to dedicate my life anew every morning as I step into the miracle of being alive one more day.

With these simple yet powerful words, I ask to be of service to others; I ask God to help me so that my own life may enhance the lives of others, may enhance the world. I don't want my presence to be exploitive or burdensome. To be humble and to be a servant is the greatest job anyone who desires liberation could have.

The earth, which includes all beings—all creatures great and small—does not belong to us. Life provides us with our greatest opportunity—to realize how we belong to the earth, how we are an intricate part of a whole. Whatever we think, whatever words we say, and whatever actions we take . . . matter to the whole. We do not exist as separate and disconnected from the rest of life, from the others who seem to appear as separate from us. When this disconnection is healed, we will come to know ourselves as we really are: holy beings.

Our lives, no matter how long, will be over before we know it. Yet we can discover the purpose of our lives if we have a sincere desire to do so, and also the willingness to accept whatever obstacles may appear in our path as opportunities to be kind and to continue on, no matter what, remembering that life is a blessing—a blessed opportunity to receive and give blessings.

THE MAGICAL POWER OF GIVING BLESSINGS

There is great power in giving blessings, not just for the recipient but also for the giver. To bless someone is to enchant them, as unconditional love is transmitted energetically from one body to another. Through blessing another you transform them into a holy being by becoming a channel for love—and in the process you become blessed, because the blessing in a psychic way moves through you first. Over time, with patience and practice, your whole world becomes populated with holy blessed beings.

Uttering the name of someone gives you tremendous power. Most people can't help but respond when their name is called. When as part of your *sadhana* you daily give a blessing along with someone's name, the specificity of the action yields positive results that over time can transform you and the people in your life into holy beings.

Here is how it works; I call it the blessing meditation. Set aside some time (morning is usually best for most people), find a comfortable seat, and sit down. Close your eyes and become aware of your breathing, breathing in and breathing out. Silently say the words "Blessings to" as you inhale, and as you exhale say the name of someone you know and love, as it is easier to give a blessing to them. Continue for several minutes, extending your blessings to include your family, friends, past boy- or girlfriends. You will find that as you say their names, their image will appear to you. With consistent practice you will be able to not only see them but also feel their presence when you name them. Over time difficult issues that you may have with them will begin to resolve; when they make an appearance in your dreams, it will

be as a benevolent positive presence. Over time you will find that when and if you do encounter them physically, your relationship with them has magically and dramatically changed—you will feel that there is a new ease in your interactions. They will seem friendlier toward you. The feeling that they are coming at you will be lessened.

No matter how many good deeds you do or how many profound and intelligent words you may speak, what people will remember most about you is how you make them feel. If you really want to live a life of service to others, it is helpful to learn ways to make others feel good. Learning how to give blessings in an anonymous way is a powerful means to transform your world and that of others. Because it is done anonymously, you don't run the risk of inflating your ego, which could happen if you were to give the blessings in person. Indeed, trying to actually contact each person every day to tell them you love them and bless them would probably prove impossible, and even become annoying. Since they live inside you anyway, the most direct means to contact them is to go within your own heart. When you say their name in a sincere loving way, you both fall into love—dissolved into the universal heart—your own true eternal being.

But don't expect immediate results. Patience is important when you are cultivating your new reality. Every action, whether it is as subtle as a thought or formed as a word or deed, is like a seed being planted in the soil that is the ground of your being. Seeds take time to grow. But it isn't only time that ensures healthy growth; a seed must also be nourished by the right foods. Consistent loving care will yield positive results. When the seeds you have planted begin to sprout, you will enjoy watching how those around you begin to blossom into the people you wish them to be. And you will discover yourself as the person you always knew you could be.

Sharon Gannon is a yoga master, author, animal activist, musician, and artist with a commitment to teaching yoga as a path to enlightenment through compassion for all beings. She is the author of several books, including *Yoga and Vegetarianism*, and cofounder of the Jivamukti Yoga Method, which is taught worldwide.

YOGA BABY

"The practice of yoga focuses on purifying the physical body, which is comprised of vibrations—of sound arising from our inner mental environment. Yoga should push you over the edge a bit. It must be physically challenging enough so you question who is the doer. Let God come in and do the work," says Sharon Gannon (who you just met).

I began studying Jivamukti yoga (my favorite form of Hatha yoga that incorporates spiritual practice and activism) with Sharon and her partner and cofounder David Life in 1992. Back then I was a dancer with lots of injuries and few solutions. A friend suggested I try yoga. Yoga? I wanted something hard-core, not gentle stretching for aging hippies. But I trusted my friend and reluctantly trucked down to a first-floor walkup in the East Village. What happened next transformed my life and planted the seeds for the self-designed healing plan I would create eleven years later when cancer came.

Roll out your mat and tend to your temple. When the great swami stretchy people created yoga, they weren't interested in a rock-hard middle or toned booty. These sages knew that the ultimate hot spot waits for us in our mind. But as you've already learned, the only way to get into the club is to meditate regularly. However, if your body is frozen and squeaky, it can be wicked painful to sit in lotus position while trying to clear your mind and focus. Let asana—yoga positions—thaw you out.

There are many forms of yoga available to us today, and each of us gravitates toward a particular style for our own reasons. Check out yogajournal.com to find a school near you and amazon.com for endless videos that allow you to have a yoga session in the comfort of your own home.

When the great swami stretchy people created yoga, they weren't interested in a rock-hard middle or toned booty.

SHAKE YOUR ASS

Of diet, meditation, and exercise, which do you think is the most important for a vibrant God pod glow? Whichever one you're not doing. Zoinks! All three are important for a well-rounded, healthy state of mind and body. The one I seem to skip the most is exercise. Lots of my gal pals have the same problem. Here's an awesome statistic I learned from Dr. Brian Clement: The body heals eight times faster when you exercise regularly. Eight times! Exercise floods the body with our favorite friend, oxygen. If you recall, lymph is circulated by a pump called move your ass! Your tissues depend on lymph to provide oxygen and carry off wastes. If the lymph doesn't circulate, then the tissues suffocate in their own acidic waste products. Gross!

Sweating is sublime. It's a perfect time to practice a new language of healthy messages sent to yourself and others. Walk and affirm positive things in your life. Dance and affirm. Fly through the air on the trapeze and affirm. "I am healthy, I am strong, I am focused, I am powerful, I am lean, I am confident, I am whole." Infuse your hip shake with the sacred spark. Sweat and reprogram! A phenomenal method to help you do this is called Intensati by Patricia Moreno. OMG! Check out her Web site, videos, and book. You will be amazed and uplifted (mind and ass cheeks). Patricia combines martial arts, aerobics, and yoga with the power of intention. Build your strength as you shout your intentions. Go to patriciamoreno.com for the deets.

The body heals eight times faster when you exercise regularly.

POUNCE ON *your bounce*

Remember the fun you had bopping on the trampoline when you were a kid? Well, today you can jump on a mini trampoline called a rebounder. Talk about fantastic cellular exercise! As you bounce, the alternation of weightlessness and gravitational pull gently squeezes your cells. This massages and stimulates the lymphatic drainage points, allowing for better elimination and increased oxygen. Rebounding boosts metabolism, improves circulation, helps digestion, and is extremely gentle on your joints.

If you're new to rebounding, try to bounce for about fifteen minutes three times a week, working your way up to thirty minutes a day, five days a week. For maximum results try breaking it up. Do fifteen minutes twice per day morning and evening. My favorite rebounder is made by Needak and costs around $250—a bargain compared with a gym membership. Rebounders are terrific if space is limited. They fold up easily and store under your bed. If your balance is wonky at first get a rebounder that comes with an optional stability bar. Keep those ankles safe, hot shot.

MOVING IS GROOVING

Get moving in whatever way works for you. Experts suggest we get our hearts pumping three to five times a week for at least thirty-five minutes. You can do that! This may seem like a big commitment, but it's not. It takes much longer to watch reality TV train wrecks while sucking back a saketini. I'll share a guilty pleasure with you. I love what I call "shit shows"—you know, the *Access Hollywood, Entertainment Tonight* gossip fests. And though I really try to limit the amount of gossiping I do myself, I can't help but tune in from time to time. Now my rule for celebrity media indulgence is simple: If I want to know who broke up with who and why they went to rehab I can only watch it while sweating on my home elliptical (perfectly placed near my flatscreen). In fact, I watch lots of films, TV shows, and documentaries this way. Before I know it, forty-five minutes have gone by and my workout was fun and highly entertaining!

Throw on your "I'm a goddess" tracksuit and start training, lady. Buy a hula hoop, install a stripper pole, gyrate to your *Flashdance* record, take up karate, round up your posse and do some double Dutch, or hit the streets or fields for a brisk walk, gentle trot, or all-out run. Some of the best workouts happen outside, in nature. Hike and bike your way through the sunshine. Fill your lungs with oxygen, your eyes with flowers, and soak in the majesty of the mother. Now, that's a workout!

YOUR *sexy* EPIDERMIS

Now that you're sweating out the toxins, let's make sure you don't lather them back on! As much as possible, you want to use natural products on your sexy epidermis. Your skin is your body's largest organ. What you put on your body, you literally absorb. So if you wouldn't drink a bottle of drugstore moisturizer, then don't put it on your body, because your skin will literally sip it in.

Today we live in a world full of substances that are potentially harmful. Because we've all been exposed to thousands of chemicals over our lifetimes, starting when we were still in the womb, we all carry many of them in our bodies. This is what's known as your body burden. How big is our body burden? According to researcher Randall Fitzgerald in his book *The Hundred-Year Lie,* pretty big.

He writes, "In 2001 scientists at the US Centers for Disease Control and Prevention in Atlanta surveyed 2,400 people and searched for 148 specific toxic compounds in their blood and urine. Every single test subject's body contained dozens of these toxins." Each toxin by itself might not be so dangerous. But what happens when you mix all these toxins together? Nobody really knows because the dangers of most of these chemicals haven't been tested alone, much less in combination.

The average consumer babe uses dozens of personal care products per day! Many of those products contain hundreds of dangerous synthetic chemical compounds. Unlike (most of) the food and drugs we ingest, the cosmetics industry requires no premarket safety tests, monitoring, or labeling. Due to massive loopholes in federal law, companies can put nearly any ingredient into your products. There's no need to be a makeup-free hippie to be healthy. These days there are many unbelievably gorgeous, nontoxic products on the market. Browse online for the latest brands that are guaranteed and clearly labeled chemical-free, natural, and organic.

Another everyday chemical hazard to stay away from are antibacterial products. Dr. Junger touched on this a bit in chapter 6, but let's take it a bit farther. Most Americans have been indoctrinated to believe that a sterile world is safer. Sure, antibacterial soaps and cleaning products kill germs—but germs are not always the enemy. And guess what? The tougher, more dangerous germs are often left behind. Overuse of antibacterial products has actually helped create the antibiotic-resistant superbugs that are now widespread. Today the antibacterial craze is expanding into everything. Triclosan, the most widely used antibacterial additive, is even found in children's toys. In fact, an Environmental Working Group study found that 97 percent of breast-feeding mothers had triclosan in their milk. Paradoxically, you'll be healthier if you're not as clean.

Kids are very susceptible to chemicals. And a lot of baby products are loaded with deadly crap. According to Campaign for Safe Cosmetics, formaldehyde and 1,4-dioxane—both known carcinogens—are used as foaming agents and can be found in more than half of children's bath soaps, shampoos, lotions, and other personal care products. To protect your kids, go with fragrance-free, pure soap products that don't have added moisturizers.

BODY BURDEN BEAUTY

with Stacy Malkan

Penis deformation? I don't like those two words together. In the Potomac River, hormone-disrupting chemicals are causing strange genital malformations in the wild kingdom—frogs, fish, and salamanders with mixed-up sex organs. In the Potomac 100 percent of male smallmouth bass are growing eggs. You read that right: Their testicles are growing eggs instead of sperm. All is not well with male genitalia in the human kingdom, either. An increasing number of boys are being born with undescended testicles and deformed penises. A quarter of American women are already contaminated with high enough levels of phthalates—plastic-softening and fragrance chemicals—to potentially cause malformations in their male offspring.

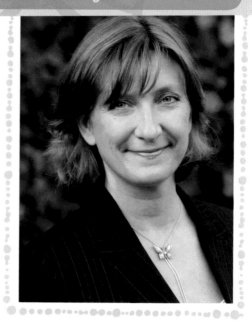

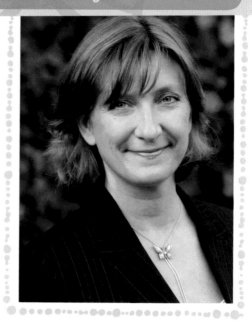

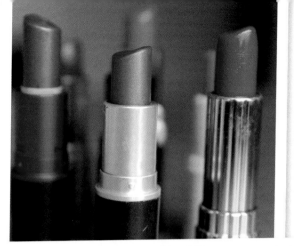

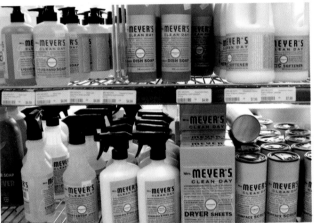

Years ago, when the Campaign for Safe Cosmetics broke the story that phthalates are found in most beauty products, more than a few people asked me: If phthalates are harmful to boys, why should we worry if they're in products used by women?

I thought, seriously? But when the question kept coming, I learned that you actually have to answer it: Um, because boys come from the bodies of women.

So yes, we need to worry about beauty products laced with gender-bending chemicals. If we want to protect boys and girls and fish and frogs, we need to keep these chemicals away from females who are, might be, or might someday want to become pregnant. We need to keep these chemicals off our bodies and out of products that run down our drains. In other words, we need to keep these chemicals out of commerce.

That's why the Campaign for Safe Cosmetics is working to pass laws to ban hazardous chemicals, and to pressure the $50 billion beauty industry to clean up its act.

In the meantime, here's what you can do to protect yourself, your loved ones, and the salamanders from exposure to hormone-disrupting chemicals:

- **AVOID PRODUCTS WITH SYNTHETIC FRAGRANCE.** Phthalates are used to make fragrances last longer. Our study found phthalates in more than 70 percent of fragrance-containing products, including shampoos, hair gels, lotions, and deodorants. None of the products listed phthalates on the label. Until we get better laws, it's best to avoid all synthetic fragrance-containing products.
- **JUST SAY NO TO COLOGNE AND PERFUMES.** There are better ways to say "I love you" than spraying gender-bending chemicals on your body!

- **CHECK LABELS CAREFULLY.** Even "fragrance-free" products may contain masking fragrances, which are chemicals used to cover up the odor of other chemicals. Choose products with no added fragrance or with natural fragrance.
- **AVOID PARABENS.** These chemicals, which can act like estrogen in the body, are used as preservatives in a wide array of lotions, shaving cream, makeup, and shower products. Avoid products that list the word parabens on the label.
- **USE EWG'S SKIN DEEP DATABASE TO CHOOSE PRODUCTS.** This free resource from the Environmental Working Group is a great way to find safer products with no parabens and no added fragrance; try the advanced search

function. It's on the Campaign for Safe Cosmetics Web site at safecosmetics.org.

- **REMEMBER THE "LESS IS BETTER" RULE.** Avoid and reduce exposures wherever you can and there will be fewer hazardous chemicals in your home, your body, and the fish. Future generations will thank you!

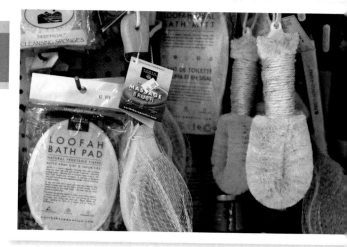

Stacy Malkan is a cofounder of the Campaign for Safe Cosmetics and author of *Not Just a Pretty Face: The Ugly Side of the Beauty Industry.*

DRY BRUSHING

Daily dry brushing is a great way to keep your skin clear of debris. Dry brushing loosens dead cells, stimulates acupressure points, tickles your chi, moves the lymph, wakes up your immune system, improves circulation, and makes your skin soft and velvety. It also reduces cellulite. Now I've gotcha!

We dump about a pound of waste from our skin on a daily basis. When your skin is clogged, those toxins reabsorb instead of being eliminated. It's normal to experience breakouts and dry patches during a detox. Your body is using the opportunity to release built-up toxins. Better out than in. It will pass, especially if you commit to helpful practices like skin brushing.

Look for a natural-bristle brush at any health food store or online. You can also use those inexpensive loofah gloves found at most drugstores. They're easy to use, plus both hands can go wild! Throw them in the wash from time to time. When using a brush, wash it with soap once a week and let it dry, otherwise it will get mildewy.

HOW TO BRUSH

Technically, experts say it's best to start with your feet and work your way up your body, using long upward strokes moving toward your heart. I like to blast Hendrix and go with my muse. It's dry

brushing, not rocket science! Throw in some circular motions (especially on your upper thighs and bum) and upward sweeps, add some shimmy, and call it a day. Pay special attention to the dimply areas.

The best time to brush is before a shower or bath in the morning. Remember to be kind, especially around your titties and other sensitive areas. Can you brush your face? Sure! Just be gentle and look for a scrubbing cloth designed specifically for that area (I just use a dry washcloth).

When I brush on a regular basis, I see a big difference in my skin. It glows. I tend to get ingrown hairs and bumps in weird places (TMI?). If I don't brush my legs, they become a highway of scales! In a nutshell, dry brushing transports me from lizard back to human—which is truly where I feel most comfortable. Make dry brushing a part of your daily beauty regime. Your temple will feel the devotion. Now go have some fun stroking yourself!

ESSENTIAL OILS

Remember the loving aromas from your grandma's kitchen or the yummy musk of your first crush? Powerful stuff. Those thought-smells always bring a smile to my face.

Close your eyes and imagine the scent of pine. Sit with that sensation, then move to peppermint, followed by lemongrass. Do you feel invigorated, uplifted, and refreshed? How about lavender or sandalwood? Relaxed? Warm? When I think of rose, I immediately feel balanced and romantic. That's because essential oils (EOs) have a positive effect on our brain, especially our hypothalamus and limbic system. Well, if your memories can bring you to that space, then imagine what your nose can do!

Your distinguished schnozz knows exactly how to harness the healing power of plants. For centuries traditional cultures have been using essential oils for purification, religious ceremonies, and medicinal purposes. Churches waft with the smell of frankincense and myrrh for a reason. And no self-respecting Buddhist would be caught dead without a stick of burning sandalwood and a strand of beads. These divine bouquets bring us two steps closer to calm and holy.

But quality is key. Remember how heat breaks down nutrients and enzymes? Well, the same holds true for therapeutic oils. Synthetic oils, those found in most "health food" stores, can be quite toxic. They're often created with solvents and high heat that damage the plants. Companies that produce synthetic oils also use chemicals to extend their

shelf life. These oils do not have the same medicinal qualities. Therapeutic-grade oils use gentle distillation methods to extract the essence of the plants. EOs are often used for their antibacterial, anti-inflammatory, hormone-balancing, and pain-reduction qualities. But most of all, EOs make ya feel happy and uplifted!

When applied topically, EOs penetrate the cell membranes, allowing them to travel through the blood and tissues in order to enhance cellular function. Because the distillation process is quite labor-intensive, an entire plant may be needed for just one drop of oil. That's why the best oils are fairly expensive.

By now you're probably anxious to find these mega potions for yourself. My two favorite brands are Essential 3 (essentialthree.com) and Young Living Essential Oils (youngliving.com). I trust their very pure products and love their blends. No matter what oil you use, make sure you spend your money wisely. Just because something smells good in the bottle doesn't mean it is good. The ingredients on the label should say "essential oil" and not "aromatherapy oil." The word "pure" should always precede the oil type (pine, cinnamon, and so on); "organic" is another quality to look for. Also do a little research and make sure the essential oils have been steam distilled, an extraction process that uses water, not chemical solvents.

HOW TO USE *essential oils*

I find these simple ways to use essential oils highly effective.

- Apply 1 to 2 drops directly to the skin to balance mood or as a perfume.
- Drink 1 to 2 drops in an 8-ounce glass of water. This is great for an upset tummy or a soothing tea. Because I encourage you to stay hydrated, EOs can be used to add a little jazz to your water intake. I particularly like adding 1 to 2 drops of lemon or grapefruit oil.
- Add 15 to 20 drops of undiluted essential oils to jojoba, avocado, coconut, or sweet almond "carrier" oil for external application. Use liberally for massage or as a healthy moisturizer.
- Inhale either directly from the bottle or through a diffuser for a lovely lift. My husband and I have a diffuser in our bedroom. When we load it up with lavender and purified water, we sleep like babies and wake up refreshed!
- Add 15 to 20 drops to a bath and soak, soak, soak (more on that later).

- For a spa-like experience or when ya have a stuffy nose, fill a bowl with hot water and a few eucalyptus oil drops. Wrap a towel around your head and bowl and let the steam open your sinuses.

You can also use oils in your cooking! I add a few drops of oregano, sage, or tarragon to a light sauté, yum! And how about dessert? Raw cacao pudding with a hint of rose or lavender! You can also add them to smoothies. Can you see key lime pie or peppermint patty? Wellness Warriors are très creative. How do ya think we keep it all going?

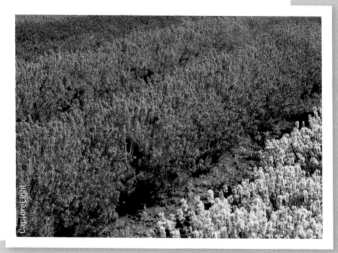

SINUS HAPPINESS

Sinus problems are one of the main reasons why people in the United States see a doctor, according to the Asthma and Allergy Foundation of America. Conventional medicines for sinus trouble—from over-the-counter antihistamines to powerful painkillers—can become harmful crutches that don't really leave you breathing easier. A neti pot, used for thousands of years by yogis and other smartypants, is a simple way to naturally and gently irrigate your sinuses with lukewarm salt water. Though it might seem like you're gonna drown the first time you use a neti pot, it's actually very easy (and refreshing!). Once you place the neti spout in your nose and tilt your noggin sideways over the sink, a gentle stream of salt water runs through your nasal passage, washing away environmental chemicals, pollen, mucus, dust, viruses, and bacteria—all the stuff your nose filters throughout the day. Make a neti cleanse part of your daily grooming ritual—wash face, brush teeth, clean nostrils. Neti pots come with instructions—using one is actually quick and easy once you get the hang of it! The folks at the Himalayan Institute (himalayan institute.org) make my favorite neti pots, salts, and washes. Great peeps.

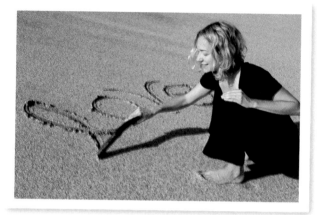

BREATH WORK

Do a body scan. Are you holding your breath right now? If so, exhale. When we're stressed, the first thing we do is shallow-breathe. Chemical sensitivity can also cause shallow breathing; so can tightness in your chest as a result of smoking, poor diet, and too much caffeine or alcohol. Perhaps you don't breathe deeply because of an old physical or emotional trauma or because in some corner of your mind a deep breath means a rounded belly and a rounded belly is "bad."

Shallow breathing can lead to a host of health problems, both physical and mental. Learning to breathe properly ensures that your body is getting all the delicious oxygen it needs. When you're breathing properly, your stomach, not your chest, rises slightly as you breathe in. When you exhale, your stomach lowers slightly. Note: Poor posture restricts the flow of air and the rise and fall of your diaphragm. So remember your mother's nagging and sit up straight!

Take some time to get frisky with your lungs. You instinctively knew how to breathe properly as an infant, but like most of us you forgot along the way. Dr. Andrew Weil has some helpful breathing how-tos on his Web site, drweil.com. Check it out! Kapalabhati breathing is another helpful technique. This yogic method is used specifically for cleansing. If you have a lot of mucus in your sinuses, it can really clear you out. Kapalabhati also helps with stress reduction and chest tension. Go to yogajournal.com to learn how to incorporate this wonderful practice into your daily life.

MASSAGE, ACUPUNCTURE, and HANDS-ON HEALING

Both massage and acupuncture are terrific for removing blockages, stimulating energy flow (chi), and creating better circulation. Plus, they help you take it down a notch.

Acupuncture—inserting very thin needles into particular points in the skin—can alleviate conditions such as headache, irritable bowel syndrome, constipation, asthma, and chronic pain. Feeling blue? Acupuncture produces a shift in the neuropeptides that control your mood. In my book, a dose of happiness and calm are well worth a little poke. But if the idea of needles makes you too queasy, try acupressure or shiatsu massage instead.

Wait. Did someone say massage? The very word calms me down. Massages are often viewed as luxury splurges. Let's change that. Your body is an instrument that must be tuned. Hands-on healing should be part of regular life maintenance. Massage gives you energy, boosts your immune system, helps your circulation, and improves the quality and quantity of your sleep. Best of all, it releases stored emotions that create issues in your tissues. There are many different types of massage that can produce lasting beneficial effects. I'll take a good deep-tissue massage any day! A few massage techniques you may not be as familiar with are craniosacral, lymphatic drainage, and Reiki.

CRANIOSACRAL THERAPY (CST)

CST restores harmony to your central nervous system through subtle pressure to the spine and cranial bones. Trained practitioners gently manipulate the cerebrospinal fluid. The peaceful and restorative massage helps with stress, migraines, and neck pain. You may be surprised at how vivid your dreams become after a treatment. Craniosacral therapy

helps me reboot my creativity when my writing tank starts running on empty.

LYMPHATIC DRAINAGE MASSAGE

You can never do too much for your lovely lymph system. Lymph massage uses light, sweeping strokes that gently move the "waters" (lymphatic fluid) toward a network of drainage points, capillaries and larger vessels studded with filters called nodes. Patients with edema may benefit greatly from lymphatic massage.

Don't be surprised if your urine smells stinky after the treatments, or if you need to whizzle more than usual. Excess fluids and toxins are simply finding their way out of your system. Drink plenty of purified water. Another great tip for keeping the fluids flowing is to avoid wearing tight-fitting bras, underpants, or hose when possible. Of course, there will be times when you feel like being a vamp or a girlie girl, so the snug and sexy stuff is okay. When you're off duty, though, let your body flow in comfy, loose cotton.

REIKI

One of the reasons I love Reiki is because I can do it to myself. Kinky! Just kidding. In Japanese, *Reiki* literally means "universal life force energy." When your life force is low, Reiki practitioners believe that you are more likely to get sick. If it's high, you're more capable of being happy and healthy. This gentle yet potent form of healing helps free energetic blockages. To understand how it works, try this: Rub your hands together vigorously for about thirty seconds. Now slowly separate your hands until they're about 2 inches apart. Feel the heat? Your hands tingle as electric impulses shoot from your palms. That's life force!

Take that energy and apply it to any neglected area in your body. You can touch it directly or let your charged hands hover about an inch or so above the pain, sadness, or dis-ease. Close your eyes and breathe deeply. Send love and release negativity. I do this when my heart aches or when I want to channel extra healing energy to my liver. Reiki is simple to learn (see reiki.com). You can give yourself or someone you love a Reiki treatment; likewise, they can give one to you.

BATHING

There's nothing quite as relaxing and luxurious as a hot, deep, and long . . . bath. At the end of a hard day at the office, on a rainy Sunday afternoon, after a day at the beach, or just about anytime at all, a soothing soak is so nice for your skin, tissues, blood flow, muscles, mind, and mood.

SAUNAS AND STEAM BATHS

Saunas and steam baths are both excellent forms of detox. The dry heat of a sauna stimulates oil-based organs, such as your liver and gallbladder. Infrared saunas are even better because the heat penetrates your tissues at a much deeper and, therefore, more cleansing level. Infrared saunas are especially good for detoxing heavy metals, chemicals, and poisons from chemotherapy or radiation treatments.

Steam heat, which is moist, stimulates and strengthens water-based organs such as your kidneys, bladder, and lungs. Just make sure your gym or spa isn't using tap water loaded with chlorine and that they keep the spaces spotlessly clean. Steam rooms can be breeding grounds for mold, mildew, and bacteria.

THERAPEUTIC BATHS

Never underestimate the healing powers of bathwater. Baths are incredibly calming and deeply therapeutic. Remember, you're a Queen (or a King),

HOT crazysexy TIP

Ginger baths are wonderful energizing soaks. Add ½ cup powdered ginger to your bathwater to induce sweat and improve circulation. You can also grate a couple of inches of fresh ginger and then squeeze it through cheesecloth (I just use my hand) to get fresh ginger juice. Note: Ginger baths are not recommended for folks with heart problems or high blood pressure.

and royal people make time for rituals. Get ye to the soul soak, Your Highness! Your adrenals will thank you.

Don't forget the candles and music, or how about a guided meditation or visualization CD? This is your time. Press pause and greet your authentic self.

Your body is a highly advanced network of storage units that holds physical, mental, and emotional power and/or pus. Remember the random stuff you'd find in your locker at the end of the school year? Old sandwiches, detention slips, a love note, perhaps a Frisbee. Your body is much like that locker. It holds the teachings (good and bad) until you're ready to release them and move on to the next school year.

Warm baths with Epsom salts and/or baking soda help remove acid waste products from your cells and tissues. Try adding 1 or 2 cups of Epsom salts, one-quarter cup of baking soda, and a dash of lavender to your bathwater. This is a great remedy for detoxing heavy metals and radiation (especially after a long flight) and helps soothe skin rashes, psoriasis, and eczema. Got a pesky hemorrhoid? Well, sit your burning ass in the tub! Epsom salt baths also reduce inflammation and relieve muscle fatigue.

Once again, let's circle back to our pH lesson. Most of your parts and pieces prefer to be slightly alkaline. Your skin is one exception. Swimming in chlorine or regular use of harsh soaps can strip your skin's acid mantle, leaving it dry and itchy. Another exception (for all you Queens out there) is your vagina. One or 2 cups of apple cider vinegar in a warm bath can help restore the proper balance. Apple cider vinegar baths also help combat unfriendly bacteria, fight fungal overgrowth, and ease the discomfort associated with vaginal and bladder infections. The next time your lady flower starts feeling funky and making bread (due to a bad diet, poor hygiene, or antibiotics) try some vinegar posthaste! Apple cider vinegar baths are also excellent for joint inflammation, arthritis, and gout.

SLEEPING BEAUTY

Lack of sleep has devastating effects on health and beauty. Once your final meal is digested, your body diverts its energy toward cleaning and repair. This happens while you catch some Zs, ideally for eight uninterrupted hours between 10 p.m. and 6 a.m. That's why it's très, très important that you finish eating three hours before going to sleep. Your body needs that precious time (and energy) to get through a long list of inner chores. When your sleep is cut short, your body doesn't have time to complete the phases needed for muscle repair, memory enhancement, the release of hormones, regulating the metabolism, and so on. If that doesn't get you motivated to snooze, this might. Lack of sleep makes you fat. According to WebMD, if you're up late, the odds are greater that you're doing some late-night snacking, which will increase your calorie intake. In addition, hormones that affect appetite take over, making you hungrier the next morning. These hormones also make you feel not as full after eating. So what do you do? You guessed it, eat more!

CREATE A SACRED SIESTA PALACE

Take a look at your sleep habits and bedroom. For optimum recharge, you want to crash out in a quiet and slightly cool environment. If your sleeping space resembles a storage unit, tidy it up, sassy. Paint it with soothing (nontoxic) colors and remove the boob tube and computer. Even the lava lamp must go! While it's fun to have sex bathed in groovy light, you want to sleep in total darkness—light leaks affect your pineal gland's production of melatonin and serotonin, the two chemicals that promote slumber.

If your budget allows, update your pillows and bedding to the organic cotton version. Research organic chemical-free mattress companies online. Sucking back flame retardants for eight hours ain't healthy. Add some plants to your room, too. Plants are nature's air purifier. Do what it takes to make your bedroom an ashram for sleeping.

Also, train yourself to sleep and rise at around the same time each day. Everyone has an internal clock, but over time and because of stress, inflexible schedules, and other modern inconveniences, we lose the ability to self-wake. Contrary to popular belief, sleep isn't something we can ever catch up on. It's okay to sleep in a bit on the weekend, but don't overdo it—you'll throw your whole rhythm off. Also, avoid stimulants like caffeine, depressants like alcohol, and strenuous exercise for a few hours before bedtime.

SNOOZING FOR ENERGY

Your good sleep intentions go straight out the bedroom window when life gets crazy (not-so-sexy) busy! Enter the nap. Our bodies have a natural rhythm of sleep and wake cycles. You've probably noticed that you feel a dip in your energy and alertness in the afternoon between about 1 and 3 p.m., even if you're well rested. That's perfectly normal—it's siesta time and your God pod knows it. If you take a nap of just twenty minutes, you'll go from feeling like a wilted plant to an alert and perky Energizer Bunny.

If it's at all possible to carve out the time for a power nap during your day, do it! All you need is a quiet place where you won't be interrupted. Empty conference rooms are a good napping spot; so is your car. A leopard-print eye mask blocks out distracting light, and a pillow and perhaps a light blanket make you comfy. Set a timer for at least twenty minutes (the alarm function on your cell is handy) and let yourself doze off. Learning to nap when you're not lying on a bed takes a little getting used to, but with practice you'll become an experienced napper, able to fall asleep quickly. Sweet dreams, beauty!

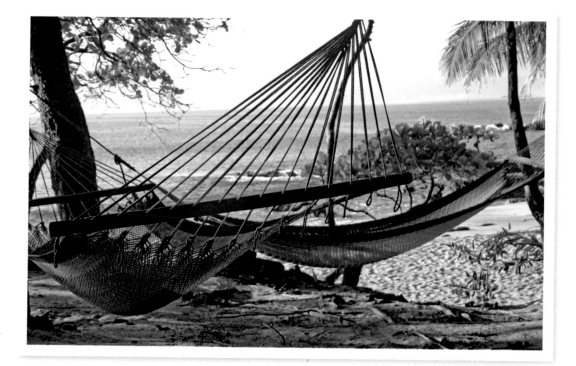

TAKE CARE

There's nothing in the least selfish or trivial about taking care of yourself. Many of us have established routines that involve gobs of the aforementioned beauty goop. Think of replacing old grooming and fitness rituals with the new ones I've outlined here. You're too pretty to pass on the chance to be even more gorgeous. When you're taking care of your body and mind, your skin and what's beneath it, you are taking care of your whole world. Why? Because, silly, when you're at your best you do your best. How nice for everyone else!

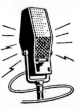

testimonial: Ana C. G.

With Kris's guidance I reconnected with my body physically, mentally, and spiritually. I'm empowered by the real energy that flows through my body as it heals naturally.

The level of energy in my body has skyrocketed. I feel clean in and out, no more toxic waste. During my first week on the cleanse I developed some detox signs that honestly scared me. I did not know what was going on until Kris wrote to expect such a reaction: rash on my arms and legs. I started dry brushing and having hot Epsom salt baths and in a few days I was me again—but better.

One thing that also helped me amazingly were some simple tools to balance and calm my body. My bath-time calming was a daily gift. Meditation guided me to my inner peace and continues to be an eye-opener for me. I had never done yoga before but today I recommend yoga to everyone. Only a few minutes a day every day helps stretch your body in a deeply satisfying way.

I also have a daily walking routine, first thing in the morning for thirty to forty-five minutes, then I do a dry brush, and oh, it's so refreshing. Now I walk for pleasure instead of just burning calories, which always felt like a torture. Feeling the morning sun on my face is an instant energizer. Wow!

CHAPTER 7 IN REVIEW

REMEMBER:

- Make and keep promises to yourself.

- Create a morning spiritual practice.

- Do nothing with purpose—learn to meditate and get into a daily habit.

- Take up a yoga practice, and try to find one taught by a true yoga master so you get both the physical and spiritual benefits from your daily routine.

- Sweat = glow.

- Many of the personal care products we use every day contain hundreds of dangerous synthetic chemical compounds.

- Charm your skin with dry brushing and essential oils.

- Take care of your sinuses with a neti pot.

- Practice breath work.

- Take it down a notch with a massage and a bath.

- Sleep, beauty . . . sleep.

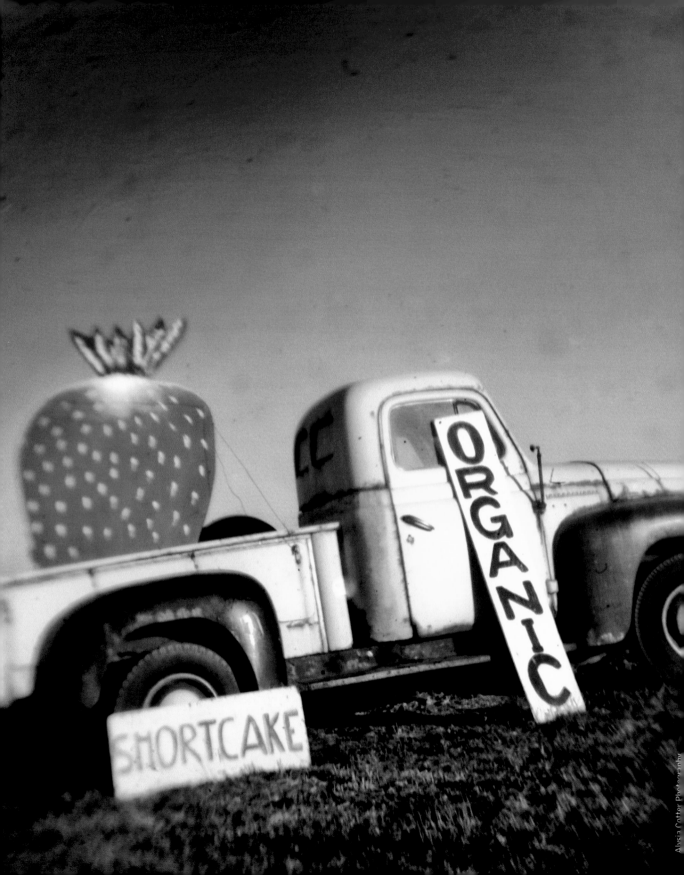

CHAPTER

8

GETTING STARTED

Feeling adventurous? Good—let's get into the nitty-gritty details of transforming your plate—and your palate. Over the next few days, embark on a sexy upgrade of your cabinets, fridge, and the shelf in the laundry room where you keep your secret vodka supply. Toss what no longer serves you.

When my pantry is stocked with a savvy stash, I'm stacked. If I open the fridge and see a jar of pickles and moldy bread—later 'gator, "We're eating out!" On the other hand, when my kitchen is ready to meet me halfway with fresh, easy-to-prepare veggies, I am inspired to browse through my cookbooks, channel my grandmother (sans the Spam cake sandwiches), and play! I love those nights. My hubby and I dine on a healthy (candlelit) homemade meal brimming with Crazy Sexy love.

TOSS IT!

First things first—clear your cupboards of crap! I know that throwing away food can generate an awful feeling of waste. But if it's bad in the first place, consuming it will be the biggest waste of all. Your body isn't a garbage can! So fear not and go forward to the compost bin: All food products, and their paper wrappers, except meat, bones, and dairy, can be added to the compost pile. Use the vodka as an astringent on your face or an antiseptic to clean a scrape.

I understand that the Toss It list can seem like a scary game of trust. You know, that cheesy corporate bonding exercise where your comrades lock arms and catch you as you fall backward (if you're lucky). Relax. If you get overwhelmed, take a deep breath and know that I will catch you, by recommending many lip-smacking treats, snacks, and veggie meals. I won't leave you lying on the conference room floor, faking a meaningful bond with the slimy dude from HR.

How does this purge fit into the 60/40 plan? If you're planning on including animal protein in your diet, make it the best you can afford, and cut back. I don't think I said anything about eating 40 percent snack cakes, toaster pastries, and salami sandwiches on white bread with mayo topped off by a double caffeinated cola. Besides, if you're ready to roll on the cleanse, temptation food has got to go—otherwise it's not a . . . drumroll . . . cleanse!

What follows is a say-sayonara refresher of those items you need to get out of your kitchen and your life:

- Acidic energy drinks, coffee, soda, diet soda, flavored chemical waters, and booze.

- All refined sugars and artificial sweeteners.

HOT crazy sexy TIP

Always, always light candles when dining. Make your meals sacred and sexy. Candlelight is flattering—no harm in looking like a starlet while noshing.

- All processed starches, especially The Whites. This includes white table salt, which is heavily processed and stripped of important minerals, white rice, white bread, and white potatoes.

- Gluten. Be a self-detective and dump it for a while—if you notice that you feel a lot better without it, keep gluten on the nevermore list. If not, remember sprouted whole grain is always best.

- Dairy. It sucks, it's gross, let it go.

- Eliminate animal foods or at the very least, reduce to no more than twice per week.

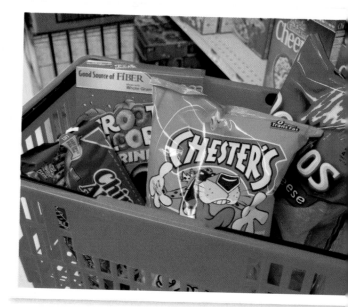

SHOP GIRL!

Done? Great! That wasn't so bad, was it? Kinda liberating, in fact. Next up, we'll create a detailed shopping list so you'll have lots of yummy foods to choose on your mission. Planning ahead saves a ton of time and money because it helps you focus and cuts down on impulse buys. Slip into your sneakers with rainbow-colored laces and get to the grocer *tout de suite!*

In the beginning, filling your cabinets with healthy essentials may seem costly. Staples such as spices, oils, and seasonings are expensive, but they also last a long time. Once you make the initial investment, your weekly bills will decrease. Remember, spending a little more upfront will help you save in the long run—especially when it comes to preventable illnesses that drain your life force and bank account!

As you stroll the aisles, keep my favorite mantras in mind:

- If it has a shelf life longer than you, don't eat it.
- If it was made in a laboratory, it takes a laboratory to digest!
- I am a Wellness Warrior, a divine banana, and I am worth this effort!

UNDERSTANDING INGREDIENTS IN OUR "FOOD" *with Stefanie Sacks*

Many supermarkets have now started using nutrition profiling systems—in the form of shelf-tag programs—to help shoppers identify healthy processed food products. What a great idea . . . not! There are several (five so far that I am aware of) different profiling systems, and each is using different criteria to determine how healthy a food is (there are no regulations for these systems as of yet). Like we weren't confused enough!

Is this going to make shopping easier for Americans? Does this mean there's no need to read ingredient lists or nutrition facts labels anymore? Or will it just make food shopping even more confusing? Because each system has different criteria, I believe it will be far more confusing for a person to navigate the grocery store.

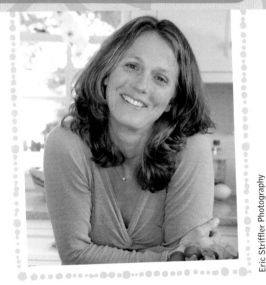

Eric Striffler Photography

My advice? When it comes to packaged food—from bags to cans and everything in between—read the ingredients and nutrition facts labels.

THE DOWN AND DIRTY ON INGREDIENT LISTS

The longer the list, the more processed the food. Choose products with the shortest lists. Keep in mind that the first ingredient listed is its main ingredient—what is most prevalent. And the last ingredient on the list? That's right—it's the one present in the smallest quantity of all. So if sugar (or some form of sugar like high-fructose corn syrup) is number one or two, the food has tons of sugar! Make sense? When it comes down to the actual ingredients, look out for the following:

ARTIFICIAL COLORS

FD&C Colors (Food Drug and Cosmetic Colors) are a wide variety of artificial colors used to color food (as well as drugs and cosmetics). Colors are typically a derivative of coal tar, a thick liquid or semi-solid tar obtained from coal. The main concerns about coal tar derivatives are that they cause cancer in animals, as well as allergic reactions. They're found primarily in processed foods (candy, confections, cereals, puddings, jelly, hot dogs, imitation foods, condiments, soft drinks, and so on). Avoid these:

- FD&C blue no. 1
- FD&C blue no. 2
- FD&C citrus red no. 2
- FD&C green no. 3
- FD&C red no. 2
- FD&C red no. 3
- FD&C red no. 40
- FD&C violet no. 1
- FD&C yellow no. 5
- FD&C yellow no. 6

Although all colors are permanently listed for use in foods and drugs with the FDA, their safety is not fully proven due to inconclusive data.

ARTIFICIAL FLAVORS/ FLAVOR ENHANCERS

There are approximately 1,500 synthetic flavorings added to foods. Most often food labels say "artificial flavors" rather than listing the individual synthetic flavorings. That's usually because the mixes of flavoring compounds are proprietary recipes. Flavor enhancers, such as monosodium glutamate (MSG), common in Chinese food and many processed soups and sauces, can cause headaches, chest pain, and numbness. Although MSG is on the list of additives needing further study, it is still considered Generally Recognized as Safe (GRAS) by the FDA. Just as MSG is GRAS, so are all of the 1,500 other synthetic flavorings.

ARTIFICIAL (AND NOT-SO-ARTIFICIAL) SWEETENERS

Artificial sweeteners refer to a group of non-nutritive, low-calorie sweeteners, all with individual properties and areas of concern. Included are:

- Aspartame
- Acesulfame K
- Neotame
- Sucralose (Splenda)
- Saccharin
- Sugar alcohols (sorbitol, xylitol, mannitol, and others)
- Tagatose

Keep a sharp eye out for high-fructose corn syrup (HFCS). Also called dextrose, this sugar is highly processed sweet syrup derived from corn (usually the genetically modified kind). It is cheaper than natural sugar. Because it's so cheap, large amounts of it are found in many, if not most, processed foods and soft drinks. HFCS is a big part of the obesity epidemic in our country, in part because it's so insidious people have no idea how much of it they are consuming.

ARTIFICIAL PRESERVATIVES

Natural preservatives include citrus (ascorbic acid), vinegar, and salt. Artificial preservatives are synthetic chemicals used to preserve food and beverages. Also Generally Recognized as Safe by the FDA, these substances do not need pre-market approval:

- Calcium propionate
- Disodium EDTA
- Nitrates/nitrites
- Potassium benzoate
- Potassium sorbate
- Sulfur dioxide
- Sodium propionate

They may not need market approval, but they need yours. Skip these additives whenever possible. A pretty long list, I know. But, put your antenna up and leave it up. Soon the label looker-outer in you will be second nature!
Source: Ruth Winter, MS, *A Consumer's Dictionary of Food Additives*

Stefanie Sacks, MS, is a culinary nutritionist practicing throughout the Hamptons and New York and vicinity. She is dedicated to helping people live healthier lives by teaching them, hands-on, how to nourish themselves through proper food choices.

crazy*sexy* SHOPPING LIST

Here's a short list of foods you'll find in my personal cache—I think they'd look good in yours, too. Some are healing staples and nutritional prize-fighters, while others are transitional foods for getting over the meaty, fatty hump. All are a diet upgrade. Again, you do not need everything! This is just a guide, a snapshot of my kitchen.

❋ VEGGIES

Your new lifestyle calls for veggies, veggies, and more veggies! They are the centerpieces of your Crazy Sexy Diet. Cucumbers, broccoli, kale, collards, celery, parsley, cabbage, romaine, red lettuce, spinach, peppers, zucchini, asparagus, red peppers, chard, green beans, alfalfa sprouts, lentil sprouts, mung bean sprouts, sweet pea and sunflower sprouts, onions, garlic, leeks, cauliflower, winter

HOT crazy*sexy* TIP

When navigating the grocery store, stay on the perimeter and avoid the middle! The perimeter is where the produce and fresh foods are found. Packaged foods are found in the middle of the store. When venturing into the inner aisles for grain, bread, and cereal, look up or down. The stuff at eye level is from big food companies that have paid big bucks for premium space. Less expensive small brands, plain old steel-cut oats, whole grains and organic pastas, and dried beans are often found below or above eye level.

squash, carrots, arugula, bok choy, sweet potatoes, parsnip, turnips . . . the list goes on! Have fun with your veggies—experiment with new tastes like kohlrabi, tat soi, and jicama. Mix and match 'em, try new seasonings, invent your own stir-fries, salads, soups, and stews. Oh, and invite me over for dinner.

✳ GLUTEN-FREE GRAINS AND NOODLES

Whole grains (gluten-free, if you're sensitive) are a big part of the Crazy Sexy approach. Good choices: millet, quinoa, buckwheat, brown rice, wild rice, amaranth, and teff as whole grains or pastas, 100 percent buckwheat soba noodles (most brands contain wheat), Tinkyada rice pasta, Ancient Harvest quinoa pasta. Oats are fine even for the gluten-sensitive or those with celiac disease, as long as they are from a safe brand (one that processes oats in equipment that does not process grains containing gluten).

✳ GLUTEN AND NON-GLUTEN BREADS AND SNACKS

Gluten-free doesn't mean bread-free or snack-free. You have lots of great choices here. Food for Life Baking Company makes yumalicious gluten-free breads and wraps. If gluten doesn't bother you, check out their sprouted Ezekiel breads and cereals. Other gluten-free products: corn tortillas, mochi, and other brown rice products. I love the brown rice crackers made by Sesmark, San-J crackers, and Edward & Sons. Check out Glutino and Glutano snacks and Pamela's Products for cookies, dessert mixes, and pancake mixes. Whole Foods makes a gluten-free line as well. Just read the labels, because some of the foods contain milk and eggs.

✳ BEANS AND LEGUMES

Chickpeas, lentils, adzuki, white beans, black beans, limas, and pinto beans are the easiest to digest.

Soak dried beans overnight in twice as much water as beans and add a $1/2$-inch strip of kombu (seaweed) to the soaking water. This helps cut down on your methane expulsion! So does discarding the soaking water and rinsing the beans before continuing on with your recipe. If you don't have the time to soak beans, Eden brand canned beans are a good alternative. Other brands contain preservatives, but Eden uses only beans, kombu, salt, and water. Rinse before using to remove up to 40 percent of the added salt.

✳ SOUP'S ON!

Fresh warm soup is a staple for people transitioning to the Crazy Sexy Diet—especially for those who live in colder climates. Make your soups tasty and hearty by using beans and a variety of veggies, especially root veggies like parsnips, celery root, yams, blue potatoes, carrots, and turnips. Add fresh herbs, lots of garlic, onion (or chives or scallions), a little olive oil, and Celtic or Himalayan sea salt. Don't worry about recipes. Just throw everything in a pot, cook until the beans and roots are tender, and season to taste. I add Pacific Foods organic vegetable broth or Rapunzel brand vegan bouillon. Miso soup is another healthy staple. Miso makes a great base for a soup with vegetables and soba noodles.

✳ FRUIT

Avocados and tomatoes (yup, technically they're fruits), apples, lemons, limes, grapefruit, pears, grapes, and berries are all good choices. While fruits are a healthy choice, low-glycemic fruits (those that are less sweet, like blueberries) are better for your blood sugar (check chapter 3 for a glycemic index refresher). Remember that fruit in general is slightly acidifying. You don't have to skip it—fruit is very cleansing, loaded with vitamins and minerals, and it makes a satisfying snack or dessert. Just go easy. Two or three servings (half a large grapefruit, one medium-size apple, a cup of berries) are plenty per day.

✳ SWEETENERS

Stevia, yacón syrup, and agave syrup are my favorite alternatives to sugar. Stevia and yacón don't affect your blood sugar; agave raises it only slightly, but not as much as sugar does. Stevia is actually an herb from a plant in the chrysanthemum family that grows in Paraguay and Brazil. Be aware that a little goes a really long way—this wonder plant is about 300 times as sweet as sugar. It comes in packets or as a liquid; brand names include SweetLeaf.

Yacón syrup is made from a tuber that grows in the Andes mountains of Peru. The syrup tastes sorta like molasses and is loaded with minerals such as potassium. Agave syrup (also sold as agave nectar) is made from the agave plant, mostly found in Mexico. It's the same plant that gives us tequila, but there's no worm in the bottle of agave syrup (dang!). Agave contains minerals such as iron and magnesium.

✳ FLOURS AND MEALS

If you can tolerate gluten in your diet, go with organic, stone-milled, whole-grain flours (stone milling preserves the bran, nutrients, and natural oils in grains). If gluten is a no-no, then you still have an amazing array of alternatives: amaranth flour, black bean flour, flaxseed meal, potato flour, oat flour, quinoa flour, millet flour, nut flour, and more. Check out Bob's Red Mill at bobsredmill.com to get an idea of what's available. Need gravy? Arrowroot and kudzu powder make terrific thickening agents.

✳ ALTERNATIVES

Cutting back or eliminating dairy products is easier than you might think. Rice, almond, oat, and hemp milk are my personal favorites as alternatives to dairy. You can make your own nut milks, too, and I'll show ya how in a hot minute.

Brooklyn-based Dr. Cow (dr-cow.com) nut "cheeses" are fabulous for special occasions, and they're probably the healthiest of all the faux cheeses on the market. You will lose your mind! Pair their cheeses with oil-cured olives and you've got yourself a really sexy hors d'oeuvre. Another good brand to know about is Eat in the Raw. They make a terrific Parmesan-like food from nuts; it's super-tasty on top of pasta, salad, and sautéed veggies. Daiya cheese is another alternative. This tapioca-based "cheese" melts like the real thing. It's great for the occasional vegan quesadillas, lasagna, and grilled cheese sandwiches. Earth Balance Natural Buttery Spread kicks dairy butter's ass! For a good mayonnaise alternative, try Nayonaise or Vegenaise. You can also make your own raw version with cashews!

✳ EGG REPLACERS

Eggs are the Elmer's glue of cooking—they make things hold together. But you can find great stand-ins in the form of soft tofu, mashed bananas, arrowroot powder, cornstarch (1 tablespoon dissolved in

HOT crazy sexy TIP

As soon as I get home I wash my veggies, let them dry, and then place them in those emerald-green lifesavers: Debbie Meyer Green Bags (greenbags.com). Bag your veggies, but skip the ties. Oxygen circulation: good for all life-forms. This helps them stay crisp longer. My hubby likes to prep the juice ahead of time—these bags make it really easy. We call them juice packets, and they're always ready to go when we want a splash of Green Goddess love! Wash and reuse the bags to cut down on planet waste.

2 tablespoons water for each egg), and chickpea flour. You'll need to experiment a bit to see what works best in different recipes. You can also try Ener-G Foods' egg replacer for baking jobs. Do stay away from processed egg substitutes meant to be low in cholesterol—these things contain egg whites and chemicals and aren't really food.

✳ MOCK MEATS

Okay, let me be honest. I think of reproduction rump roast, tofu-turkey, and other pretend meats as methadone for tush eaters who are trying to quit the carnivore habit. This stuff is highly processed, and too much of it defeats the purpose of living a veggie lifestyle. However, some mock substitutes are healthier than others, and if you are having trouble transitioning, meat substitutes serve a valuable purpose. They get you over the hump, or in this case, the rump (roast). Here are my favorites:

- Gardein (gardein.com) is a dynamic new company that makes wonderful meat-like products (though they do contain gluten). Gardein makes everything from buffalo wings to beef skewers. My personal favorites are the Chick'n Scallopini and beefless tips.

- Sunshine Veggie Burgers (sunshineburger.com) are wheat-, gluten- and soy-free, and delicious. Gardenburgers (gardenburger.com) are a great brand as well, but read the package carefully. A few of their products contain dairy.

- Field Roast Grain Meat Company (fieldroast.com) makes yummy grain-based "meats" including sausages, cutlets, and even holiday meat loaf. Their smoked-apple sage sausages are delish.

- Check out Lightlife brand (lightlife.com) for tasty tempeh bacon, and use their Gimme Lean to make outstanding mock meatballs. Isa Chandra Moskowitz has a fabulous recipe in her cookbook, *Veganomicon* (also included in my resources section).

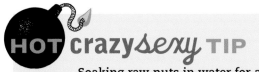

HOT crazysexy TIP

Soaking raw nuts in water for a few hours makes them more digestible; it removes the natural enzyme inhibitors that keep them from spoiling.

- Morning Star Chik'n Strips (morningstarfarms.com) are pretty darn fabulous too, especially on a Caesar salad. They do contain some gluten.

As much as possible use soy products that are close to their whole form. Soybeans, edamame, tempeh, and moderate amounts of tofu are your best choices. And if you're down on soy altogether, don't fret! There are many wonderful raw, nut-based meat-substitute recipes out there as well.

✳ NUTS AND SEEDS

Nuts and seeds are an important part of the Crazy Sexy Diet. These little gems are packed with vitamins, minerals, good fats, protein, and fiber. Your options include: almonds, pecans, walnuts, macadamias, hazelnuts, pine nuts, pumpkin seeds, flaxseed (use a small grinder for these or buy them already ground), sesame seeds, hemp seeds, chia seeds (these make yummy cereal and puddings), and sunflower seeds. For spreads, try raw almond butter, cashew butter, and tahini (made from sesame seeds). Always buy fresh raw nuts and store them in the fridge or freezer; roasted nuts go rancid much more quickly.

Peanuts and peanut butter can be kinda sketchy. The plants are usually heavily sprayed with pesticides. Even organically grown peanuts can harbor mold, including dangerous kinds that give off toxins called aflatoxins. If you enjoy peanut butter, buy organic, and eat it in moderation.

✱ SEASONINGS

Fresh and organic seasonings are best, but dried herbs are fine, too. My staples are pretty simple: Celtic or Himalayan sea salt, Herbamare (sea salt and herbs), dulse flakes, wheat-free tamari, Bragg's Liquid Aminos, ginger powder, garlic powder, basil, parsley, cilantro, mint, dill, rosemary, thyme, black pepper, curry, turmeric, cinnamon, cayenne, mustard seeds, and wasabi. Spice Hunter (spicehunter.com) makes fun blends. My favorite is a peppy, salt-free mixture called Zip. Pumpkin spice and apple pie seasoning, vanilla bean, or alcohol-free vanilla extract are great to add to smoothies.

✱ FERMENTED FOODS

Naturally fermented foods such as raw (vinegar-free) sauerkraut and kimchi are high in good bacteria; they're also a good source of B vitamins. They must be raw, however. Pasteurization kills life (good and bad), destroys enzymes, and reduces the nutrient content. Another reason a plant-based diet loaded with complex carbs and raw fruits and veggies is so great for you is that their fibers act as prebiotics. Prebiotics are the food your probiotic bacteria dine on. This nourishment makes them strong and healthy, allowing them to multiply and keep their king-of-the-roost status in your colon. Valuable fermented foods include Bragg's organic unpasteurized apple cider vinegar, tempeh, raw sauerkraut, and unpasteurized white miso (awesome in dressings, spreads, and soup). Nutritional yeast gives dishes a cheesy flavor—it's a lovely substitute for Parmesan. Nutritional yeast is the only form of yeast that I use in cooking and prepping. It's not the same as the yeast used to make bread and shouldn't be a problem if you're dealing with candida.

✱ SEAWEED

Seaweed is loaded with minerals and flavor. I especially love to make raw or cooked nori rolls, a mouthwatering mineral delight. Here's another great tip: Plop leftover veggies and grains on a nori sheet, wrap, and zoom. Popular seaweeds include dulse (great on top of salads), arame, hijiki, and wakame (add this one to miso soup).

✱ DRINKS

My favorite replacements for soda, sugary pasteurized juices, coffee, and other drinks are purified water with lemon, herbal teas, green tea, white tea, yerba maté, kukicha, chai, kombucha, and coconut water. Fruit water is also delicious. Toss purified water and one piece of fruit with a dash of stevia in your blender. Blend and strain. Add ice. Yum! My favorite is strawberry with a mint sprig (sometimes I add a splash of sake—shhh, it's our secret!).

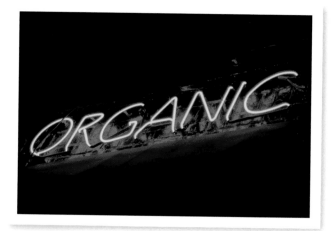

HOT crazy sexy TIP

Nutritional yeast is a good source of protein and many brands are fortified with vitamin B_{12}. Add it to your food—atop air-popped popcorn, salads, pasta, veggies—you name it! Nutritional yeast is found in the bulk food or supplement section of most health food stores.

GOOD SNACKS, CHOCOLATE, AND EASY CHOW

You'll be amazed at all the great snack foods you can eat on the Crazy Sexy Diet. Stuff like brown rice cakes, flax crackers, fresh salsa (made with lemon or lime juice), hummus, guacamole, Guiltless Gourmet tortilla chips, oil-cured olives, and air-popped popcorn are all easy to find in the supermarket or make yourself. For emergency snacking and last-minute meals, I like organic veggie burritos and cheese-free pizzas from Amy's Kitchen (amyskitchen.com). Chocolate bars, anyone? Dagoba (dagobachocolate.com) and Green & Black's (greenandblacks.com) are two high-quality, affordable, and tasty brands. Carob is also a terrific choice, especially because it doesn't contain any caffeine. Goldie's Carob Bars (goldies carobbars-ny.com) are my personal favorite. How about something creamy and dreamy like ice cream? Check out Turtle Mountain (turtlemountain.com) Purely Decadent coconut milk ice cream and Luna and Larry's (www.coconutbliss.com) organic coconut bliss ice cream. They're so good I could roar!

RAW AND LIVE TREATS

Once you start exploring raw foods, you'll run across some really tasty raw snacks. For a good variety

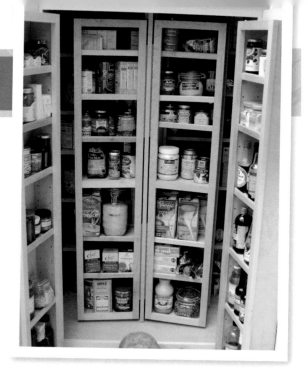

of fun raw food products, check out Lydia's Organics, Foods Alive crackers, Lärabars, Just Tomatoes dehydrated veggies, and Ruth's Hemp Foods (they make a great chia cereal, too). Products from Glaser Organic Farms are out of this world. I love their chickpea carrot croquettes and raw brownies. UliMana raw chocolate truffles (OMG!), Kookie Karma's yummy raw cookies, and delish raw nut-based ice cream made by my pals at Organic Nectars are all a must!

GOOD FATS ARE FOXY

Every woman I know needs serious fat rehab. Fat is not the enemy, ladies (and gents). Sexy people eat healthy fats! The low-fat, fat-free craze made us rounder and turned fats into the Freddy Krueger of foods. Dump that nonsense and replace it with the mantra: Nothing tastes as good as healthy! And

HOT crazysexy TIP

It's best to buy oils packaged in dark bottles and to store them in a cool dark place—this keeps them from oxidizing and going rancid.

in order to be healthy, your sizzling body needs a moderate amount of good fats. (Just don't go overboard.) Got it? Fantastic!

Good fats assist in the absorption and transport of vitamins. They increase your metabolism and can actually help us lose weight in the process! Good fats are necessary for a strong immune system, hormone production, strengthening cell walls, joint lubrication, organ protection, a healthy nervous system, and proper brain function. In fact, it's hard to be a smarty-pants without good fats. A high-functioning happy brain is partly a result of the quantity and quality of fat you eat.

Bad fats—saturated and partially hydrogenated or trans fats—are the hip and health busters. If you'd prefer to avoid clogged arteries and cottage cheese thighs, then stay away from bad fats, fried fats, and fake fats.

Read the label on a package of just about any processed food, even frozen pizza, and you'll see something called partially hydrogenated vegetable oil. Vegetable oil—that's good, right? Not when it's been heavily processed under high heat and pressure to make it partially hydrogenated, which is just another way of saying it's been turned into trans fats.

When trans fats are manufactured, the fat molecules become distorted into shapes your body can't even recognize as food. These nasty molecules create inflammation, cardiovascular harm, liver, kidney, and bowel stagnation, and an accelerated aging process. In short: Trans fats are a bitch. They're so ugly that in 2006 New York City banned the use of trans fats in restaurants. Since then, many food manufacturers and restaurant chains have followed suit. Join them. Stay away from margarine and shortening (aka trans fats), commercial cooking sprays, and other heavily processed vegetable oils such as corn, canola, and peanut oil. They all wreak havoc on your system.

CHANGE YOUR OIL

Be Italian! Match up organic cold-pressed extra-virgin olive oil with your veggies and let them make love. Flaxseed oil, hemp seed oil, walnut oil, and Udo's Choice (a blend of healthy oils) are sexy sweethearts, too. They're loaded with healthy omega-3 fatty acids—important for memory, reducing inflammation, and lots of other good stuff. More great salad oils include macadamia nut oil and avocado oil.

For cooking, choose olive oil (but use low heat), sesame, grapeseed, and coconut oil. Though technically a saturated fat, in a moderate amount coconut oil is terrific for you. It gets a bad rap when turned into a partially hydrogenated trans fat. But in its natural and unrefined form, coconut oil is healing and delicious. It's about 50 percent lauric acid, the same wonderful substance found in breast milk, and boosts immunity.

Young Thai coconut meat is great, too. It's loaded with good fats and many nutrients. Coconut water is also a fantastic source of electrolytes, and coconuts boost metabolism and have antiviral and antifungal properties. Add them to your smoothies and look out, world!

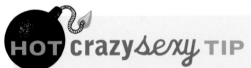

HOT crazy sexy TIP

Cooked oil is a source of free radicals. When cooking, make sure you use oils that are meant for medium to high heat, such as grapeseed oil or coconut oil. Or skip the heated oil altogether—do a water sauté or steam, and then add your oil afterward for flavor and nutrition. Certain oils like flaxseed and hemp seed are far too heat-sensitive and should never be used for cooking.

crazysexy KITCHEN EQUIPMENT

Wellness Warriors don't use swords.
Instead, we fight with kitchen equipment! In addition to a good blender and juicer (check back to chapter 6 for recommendations), place the following essentials on your wish list.

✳ SLICING TOOLS

Spiralizers and Saladaccos are nifty gadgets that turn a big zucchini (or sweet potato or whatever) into spaghetti-like strands in about thirty seconds. Swap out the blades for slicing or grating. Ditto for a traditional mandoline slicer, which is fabulous for raw lasagna recipes.

Food processors rock! I love the Cuisinart, but any heavy-duty brand will do. Use a food processor for prepping ingredients that require a fine chop but still rely on some texture. A fast way to prep a salad is to use your greens as a base and then slice up a bunch of veggies in your food processor to top.

✳ KNIVES

Good knives are the foundation of any kitchen. Select brands and sizes that suit your gorgeous hands and keep them sharp. My favorites are made by NHS, a Japanese company. Their rectangular-shaped vegetable knife is awe inspiring! You may also want to invest in a cleaver for opening coconuts. Just watch your digits, cutie.

✳ COOKWARE

Please avoid using Teflon or other nonstick cookware—the nonstick lining is a carcinogen and can come off into your food at high temperatures. I like cooking in stainless-steel pots and pans. Clay pots and cast iron are good, too. Also—though they're not cookware items per se, but small appliances—it's best to avoid microwaves. Too many researchers and scientists have studied the process food goes through when it's microwaved to make me feel comfortable about using one in my home. For instance, Dr. Hans Ulrich Hertel, now retired, worked as a food scientist with one of the major Swiss food companies that do business on a global scale. He found that microwave cooking degraded food. Other researchers have found similar results in controlled studies: Microwaves changed food's nutrients so that changes took place in the participants' blood that could cause deterioration in human systems. No thanks!

✳ COFFEE GRINDER

Lay off the java, but save that grinder. It's great for grinding spices, nuts, and seeds.

✳ NUT MILK BAG

Making your own nut milks is easy and saves a lot of money over buying prepared brands. Here's how it works: Place 1 cup of soaked nuts in the blender with 2 cups of purified water. Whirl until smooth. Pour the mixture into a nut milk bag and squeeze! You can also grow sprouts in these bags, which is why they're often sold under the name sprout bags. A down-and-dirty nut milk recipe goes something like this: 1 tablespoon of raw almond butter, 1 to 2 cups of purified water, stevia, vanilla, and cinnamon to taste. Ya don't even need the bag for that one!

✳ FOOD DEHYDRATOR

This machine is optional, but food dehydrators allow you to make fancier raw cuisine and are really helpful if you have a vegetable garden or belong to a community-supported agriculture (CSA) farm.

They're also great if you have kids—for some reason they love watching vegetables dry. Once dehydrated, surplus veggies can be stored and enjoyed for quite some time. Excalibur makes a good one that's easy to use.

✴ VACUUM SEALER

If you plan to freeze fresh local food for out-of-season use, I recommend a vacuum sealer. Air is the enemy of food in the freezer. It causes freezer burn, deterioration, and nutrient loss. FoodSaver's MealSaver Compact Vacuum Sealing System is a sturdy, affordable machine.

✴ ADDITIONAL GADGETS

Other essentials for the Crazy Sexy kitchen include a salad spinner, strainer, vegetable peeler, measuring cups and spoons, garlic press, spatulas, large

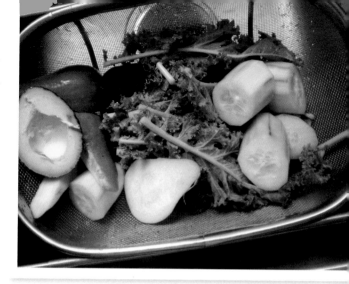

salad bowls, large cutting board, and glass mason jars with lids. I like to use the latter to store grains and to carry juice. Stainless-steel containers are a great way to tote water but get kinda stinky with juice.

CUTTING COSTS

A mostly raw, organic lifestyle costs a bit more—or maybe not. Look at what you would likely spend if you ate three meals a day at the popular drive-through feeding trough known as McDonald's.

Even though I'm not a big fan of counting calories, that works out to about 2,200 calories, about 400 more calories than the average adult woman needs. I can certainly eat very well, and quite healthfully, for $19.70 per day, especially if I lovingly prepare the food myself. Plus, eating out takes a toll on me, even when it's good food. Simple Kris-style food makes the healing difference for my God pod. It's easy, it's cozy, and it's all yours.

Breakfast:

Egg McMuffin	$2.40
Medium OJ	$1.70
Large coffee	$1.50

Lunch:

Big Mac	$3.80
Medium fries	$1.55
Medium iced tea	$1.40

Dinner:

Premium Salad with chicken	$4.95
Oatmeal raisin cookies	$1.00
Medium Coke	$1.40

Total: $19.70

SUPPORT YOUR LOCAL FARMERS

Farmers' markets and farm stands are a great way to get the freshest fruits, veggies, and other locally grown products. Not every small farmer has done all the piles of paperwork necessary to be "officially" organic, but that doesn't mean they aren't—many use sustainable methods. Do a little research so that you feel confident that the food isn't full of artificial fertilizers, insecticides, and hormones.

If you get to the market first thing, you'll have the best choices—but if you wait until the last half hour or so, you'll get the best bargains. Packing up is a drag, so the farmers are usually willing to haggle (a blood sport in my family).

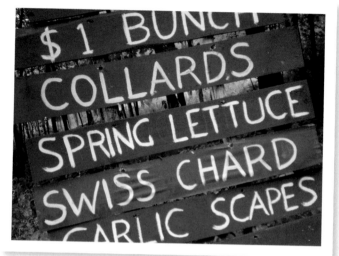

BUY THE FARM

Well, not the whole thing, just a sweet little piece of it. I followed in my mom's high-heeled steps and joined a nearby farm offering community-supported agriculture (CSA). Why? Because when I asked the lady at the CSA farm how many cucumbers I could have, she said, "As many as you want." I nearly orgasmed (in front of my mom, which was . . . awkward)! "As many as I want? Mom, get the truck!" Since I juice about twenty-one-plus cukes per week, CSAs are better than Christmas, better than Saks!

Your CSA share buys you tons of peas and peace for months. And you don't just get the standards. Unusual chlorophylls, like garlic scapes and kohlrabi, are abundant. Flowers, too! Here's how it works: You buy an advance share of the produce the farmer plans to grow. When the crop starts coming, you swing by the farm and pick up your share on a designated day. It's just amazing what a share gets you. In fact, your portion might be too much to get through. If that's the case, find someone to go halfsies.

Want to find a CSA farm near you? Ask at the local farmers' market and farm stands, and also check localharvest.org, a great Web site for tracking down CSAs and local farms.

YOU GROW GIRL!

If you really want to know where your food is coming from, grow it yourself. It's surprisingly easy to sprout your own beans, grow your own wheatgrass, and raise an herb garden on a windowsill. Tomatoes, cukes, zucchini, lettuce, herbs—they'll grow like crazy on a patio or on that favorite urban perch, the fire escape. If you have a yard, consider turning part of it into a Crazy Sexy victory garden.

Think of it this way: A packet of cucumber seeds costs about two bucks. Plant just half the packet (unless you want them to take over your neighborhood), water, give them an old piece of trellis to climb, and about forty days later you'll see tons of cukes. Not bad for a buck. Even a small garden can give you hundreds of dollars of produce each season for very little investment. Plus, you save money on your gym membership. Pushing a wheelbarrow really tones the ass!

FROSTED FOLLIES

Another big money saver is buying frozen veggies and fruits (or vacuum sealing and freezing your overflow from the CSA). Because these foods go straight from field to frozen right after picking, they can actually contain more nutrients than the fresh versions that have spent a week (or more) in transit on their way to the store. Look for organic brands (Cascadian Farm is widely available in conventional supermarkets) for frozen berries for smoothies and frozen veggies for soups, stews, and casseroles.

BULK UP

Buying in bulk is one of the best ways to save. Warehouse clubs like Costco and Sam's Club now carry a lot of organic produce, and the prices are very good. Okay, these stores are big corporate monsters, but when the farmers' market is closed for the winter, they're the way to go. Plus, when you buy organic at these behemoths, it sends an important message. Organic food rules! The package sizes are large, but you can always freeze what you don't use or share it with a pal. If you have time to volunteer, food co-ops are another good way to save through bulk buying. To locate one, go online or ask around at the health food store.

HOT crazy sexy TIP

Try to shop several times per week (around two or three visits). This way your veggie supply won't spoil if Lady Gaga suddenly invites you to Europe. Creative smoothies or blended soups mop up the extra produce that would otherwise go bad. Be thrifty, lady. Would it be more fun to use exactly what you want when you want it? Duh, of course! Sometimes I find myself going to the store because I'm missing a specific ingredient, but I'll come out with $50 worth of other stuff that "I might as well get while I'm here." If I could resist the urge, I'd be forced to use the wonderful foods I already have.

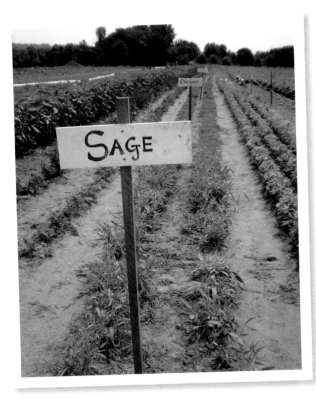

GETTING THE BEST FROM
CONVENTIONAL FOODS

Of course, we all want to buy only organic, but that's not always possible. Fortunately, not all your fruits and veggies need to be organically grown to be relatively safe. Wash all conventional veggies well. You can also soak them in a little white wine vinegar or food-grade hydrogen peroxide (you can buy this online or at the health food store—it's not the same as the hydrogen peroxide sold in the pharmacy, do not use that!). Since agricultural chemical sprays stay on the surface of the food, be sure to peel certain produce to remove any residue. Check out the following advice to guide you.

THE DIRTY DOZEN AND THE CLEAN FIFTEEN

When buying veggies on a budget, choose the conventional option from the Clean Fifteen and try to go organic for the Dirty Dozen. What's that? It's a handy list put together by the Environmental Working Group (EWG) that will educate you on produce grown with the least and the most amount of pesticides. Here's the list of worst offenders and best choices:

THE *dirty* DOZEN

Foods grown with the most pesticides, ranked from worst to less bad

1. Peach
2. Apple
3. Bell pepper
4. Celery
5. Nectarine
6. Strawberries
7. Cherries
8. Kale
9. Lettuce
10. Grapes (imported)
11. Carrot
12. Pear

For more information about the list, check the EWG's Web site at foodnews.org or ewg.org.

THE *clean* FIFTEEN

Foods grown with the least amount of pesticides, ranked from best to not-so-good

1. Onion
2. Avocado
3. Sweet corn
4. Pineapple
5. Mango
6. Asparagus
7. Sweet peas
8. Kiwi
9. Cabbage
10. Eggplant
11. Papaya
12. Watermelon
13. Broccoli
14. Tomato
15. Sweet potato

EATING OUT

with Kathy Freston

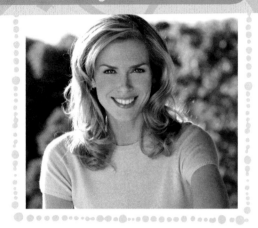

If you're eating out, there are countless restaurants that cater to vegetarians and vegans. Vegcooking.com features regional vegetarian restaurants, restaurant chains that offer vegetarian options, and links to other Web sites that list vegetarian-friendly eateries. Ethnic restaurants, especially Thai, Indian, Ethiopian, Chinese, and Mexican, are always a good choice, as they offer a variety of vegetarian and vegan options.

If you're still looking for a burger and fries, many chain restaurants, including Johnny Rockets, Denny's, and Ruby Tuesday's serve veggie burgers. Just don't drive yourself—and your dining companions—crazy worrying that your veggie burger was prepared on the same surface as the hamburgers. It might be a bit aesthetically troublesome, but it won't harm animals (or the planet) if your food is cooked on the same grill as meat. Unless you absolutely can't stomach it, let it pass.

Vegans and vegan wannabes, I believe that when you're eating out, you also shouldn't be too concerned about ingredients that make up less than 2 percent of your meal. You'll obviously want to avoid dishes served with meat, cheese, or eggs, but it doesn't really matter if there's a modicum of butter or whey or other animal product in the bun that your veggie burger is served on.

You won't stop animal suffering by avoiding such minuscule amounts of animal ingredients. But you may give your nonvegan friends—not to mention the restaurant wait staff—the idea that vegans are difficult to please. The goal is to show others how easy it is to eat in an animal-friendly manner and that restaurants can satisfy vegan customers without having to do cartwheels. I understand the desire to eliminate every last bit of animal ingredients from your diet, but let's face it: Even vegan foods cause some small animals to be tilled during farming. (Note: Since more than 70 percent of all grain, soybeans, and other crops are fed to farmed animals, not to humans, there is a lot more tiller death in chicken, turkey, pork, and beef than in plant foods, but the point should still give vegetarians a bit of humility.)

Vegetarianism is not a personal purity test. Our positive and reasonable influence on others is just as important as our own commitment to a conscious and compassionate diet.

Consider your choices: heart disease, colon cancer, plus-size pants, melting ice caps, gale-force storms, and animal suffering versus good health, energy, a trim physique, a livable planet, compassion, and tasty, diverse foods. It's clear that going vegetarian or vegan is an excellent choice as we move toward living a more conscious life.

Kathy Freston is a health and wellness expert and best-selling author of *Quantum Wellness*.

EATING SANELY

If every dazzling person would make just a few changes, just think how much healthier we could be. Our planet would thank us; the animals would lick us. That's the goal, my friend. Do the best you can and if you stumble, don't marinate in guilt. Get back on the shiny wagon and start anew. Also, don't break your bank trying to get healthy. Slowly upgrade and add as finances allow. Life is too sweet to be bitter, so just do your best. No beating, anxiety, or neurosis, por favor.

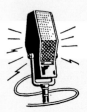

testimonial: Michelle D.

Recently I went to a naturopath out of desperation because I had been living with tummy trouble for five years, since my diagnosis of juvenile diabetes, and no MD seemed able to help me. I soon realized that although what I was eating was healthy by SAD standards, I had changes to make. Evolution, not revolution: It has been a gradual process. In the last year I've been almost vegan. The support and information I have received from Kris's Web site, crazysexylife.com, has helped me to solidify that commitment. I feel like veganism is necessary for my physical as well as spiritual and emotional health. During her cleanse I gave up the occasional chicken and fish I had continued to consume every week or so, added in more salads and other raw food, stopped making (and craving) sweets, and finally began to use my juicer.

Although I had already been doing green smoothies every morning, and eating a plant-based diet, this fine-tuning led to some detoxing. I was surprised to get symptoms like headaches and pimples, since I thought my diet was already so clean! It just goes to show how sensitive our systems are, and how they need all the help they can get. The Crazy Sexy Diet has helped me to better understand the importance of being alkaline, fighting disease with nutrition, and living the very best, most vibrant life I can.

CHAPTER 8 IN REVIEW

REMEMBER:

- Clean the crap from your cupboards and learn to shop smart. Even a 60/40 diet means high-quality food!

- Get to know your Crazy Sexy shopping list, crammed full of produce, grains, beans, nuts, seeds, seasonings, fermented goodies, great fats, and much more.

- Stock your kitchen with the right tools to make meal prep a snap—and fun, too.

- Get cozy with your greengrocer, farmers' market, and local food co-op.

- Grow your own grub—at least an herb garden or a patio tomato. Even city girls can raise wheatgrass and basil.

- Familiarize yourself with the Dirty Dozen and Clean Fifteen.

- Eat out with ease—don't be a bore, but do make the right choices without fanfare.

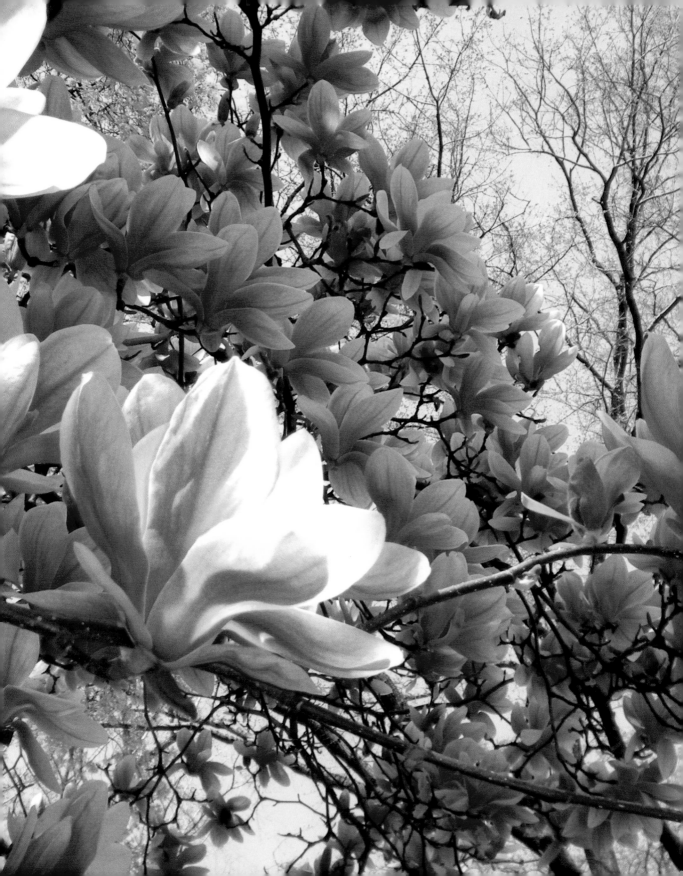

crazysexy SUPPLEMENTS

As we've been yakking about for the past several chapters, it's best to get nutrients—vitamins, minerals, enzymes, oxygen, phytonutrients—from a whole, organic, plant-based diet. Yet there are healthful ways to augment and enhance your existing diet with what I call the foundationals. These are basic products (supplements, superfoods, protein powders) that boost your diet and your health. Make no mistake—supplements and pills are not food replacements, they are diet enhancements. They complement what you are doing in your diet!

What follows are my faves, but they're just suggestions, along with explanations as to how these extras work in partnership with your Crazy Sexy Diet. For more information on foundational supplements, go to the crazysexylife .com store. We're always updating with our favorite brands!

When shopping for supplements, buy the very best quality you can afford. There is a difference between mass-produced synthetic vitamins that have been sitting on the shelf at the drugstore for six months and smaller-batch brands made with fine organic ingredients that come from whole foods. To tailor a supplement and superfood plan specific to you, however, it's a good idea for you to see a holistic doctor or naturopath for a customized plan.

PROBIOTICS

Let's be real here: Sometimes your friendly bacteria could use a hand, such as when you don't make the best food choices thanks to circumstances or desire, or you need to take drugs (maybe antibiotics) for an illness, or you undergo treatment like chemotherapy. That's why the first foundational I recommend is a good probiotic supplement—a supplement that contains beneficial bacteria by the billions and can help restore the balance in your intestines. Literally meaning "for life," probiotics are supplements containing zillions of dormant little bacteria, and they are taken to maintain or restore the body's proper bacterial balance.

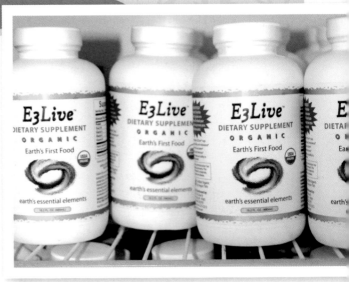

You'll notice that the probiotics shelf is a big one in most health food stores today—they've caught on. How can you choose among all the different brands and claims? What you want are bacteria that give off lactic acid as a by-product of their metabolism. (Trust me, this is a good thing.) Lots of beneficial bacteria do this, including various strains of bifidobacteria, boulardii, acidophilus, and lactobacillus. Some brands have fructo-oligosaccharides, or FOS, added to them—these are natural sugars that help feed the beneficial bacteria and get them started in your small intestine. You can also find brands with added vitamins, minerals, amino acids, and other supplements.

No matter what brand you choose, look for one high in lactobacillus and bifidobacterium. The count should be in the billions (yes, billions with a *b*). In addition, choose those that are vegetarian and come in an enteric-coated capsule. The coating keeps the bacteria safely inside until the capsule leaves your stomach and enters your small intestine. Today most probiotics brands don't need to be refrigerated—good for me, as I travel a lot. Dr. Ohhira's is

A NOTE ON *antibiotics*

Sometimes it just can't be avoided—an antibiotic becomes necessary when you have an infection that just won't go away on its own. The problem is, many antibiotics are overprescribed and become ineffective against the bugs they're supposed to fight and kill. Ever-stronger versions are required, and meanwhile those buggies react by creating new, stronger forms of antibiotic-resistant "superbugs." If you do have to take a course of antibiotics, take all the pills. Because antibiotics kill both good and bad bacteria in your intestines, when you're done with the prescription, follow up with probiotics to restore the balance of good bacteria.

one such great brand. I also like Jarrow Formulas and PB8 brands. For just keeping things in balance, one or two capsules a day should be enough. If your intestinal flora are way off, you may need to take larger daily doses, possibly for several weeks or longer. Consult with a naturopath or integrative MD if you sense a bigger imbalance. They can order a comprehensive digestive stool analysis to see if you have an imbalance between good and bad bacteria.

SUPERFOODS and PROTEIN POWDERS

A superfood is one especially rich in phyto-chemicals (natural and unique plant chemicals that have disease-fighting properties). Phytochemicals can reduce the risk of certain forms of cancer, reduce inflammation, strengthen the immune system, and in general contribute to a healthier more fab you.

Blue-green algae (BGA) harvested from Upper Klamath Lake in Oregon are a top superfood. E3Live (e3live.com) is a great brand. BGA provide a boost in energy and mental clarity, rebuild cells, and bind free radicals; they're also high in vitamins and minerals.

Spirulina is a type of algae that's high in chlorophyll and protein. Nutrex Hawaii (nutrex-hawaii.com) has a good spirulina called Hawaiian Pacifica.

Chlorella is another type of algae that helps raise pH levels, normalize bowel function, build your immune system, and bind heavy metals and radiation. If you have elevated levels of mercury (possibly from amalgam dental filings) or other environmental toxins, make chlorella your new BFF. Check out the Sun Chlorella brand at sunchlorellausa.com.

Green powders usually contain mostly dehydrated cereal grasses, such as wheatgrass and kamut. They should be used as a supplement, not in place of juicing. I love Amazing Grass brand (amazinggrass.com). You can toss a spoonful into your juice or a smoothie. Hemp powder is high in protein, and raw cacao and carob powders add antioxidants and flavor to smoothies. Nutiva (nutiva.com) has great hemp powder and seeds. Vegan triathlete Brendan Brazier's Vega brand (sequelnaturals.com/vega) is another high-quality protein powder choice. So is Sun Warrior Protein (sunwarrior.com). They also make a green powder.

Browse superfood products made by Navitas (navitasnaturals.com). The company's maca powder is great for the adrenals and sex drive. I won't tell you how I know it helps. . . . MSM (methylsulfonyl-methane) is a safe, natural, side-effect-free remedy for many types of pain and inflammatory conditions. MSM, also known as the beauty mineral, helps to create thick hair, clear soft skin, and strong nails. It also helps the tissues become more permeable, allowing nutrients to absorb and pass through while toxins move out. Rich's brand makes a good product.

DON'T WORRY, B HAPPY!

There's only one vitamin you really need when you switch to an animal-free diet: B_{12}. That's because vitamin B_{12} isn't found in plant food. It's naturally produced by microorganisms in soil and water that hasn't been contaminated or chlorinated. Animals eat unwashed plants and soil particles and drink water containing the organisms that make B_{12}, but we don't. Since you can't make it in your body and you don't get it from a vegan diet, you need to supplement. Just 2.4 micrograms per day will ensure you are getting what you need. It is the smallest daily requirement of any supplement.

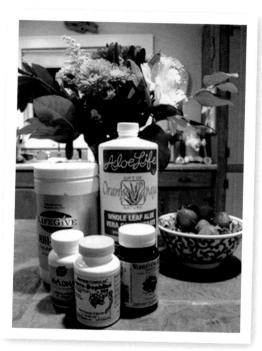

Many nutritionists recommend taking a complete B vitamin supplement, which contains other members of the B family, such as folic acid (crucial for women of childbearing age). If you prefer to take only B_{12}, sublingual lozenges dissolve under your tongue and the B_{12} gets absorbed straight into your bloodstream. Whichever way you go, choose a product that contains the B_{12} in the form of methyl-cobalamin—you absorb this best.

VITAMIN D

You need vitamin D for strong bones and a strong immune system. There's plenty of evidence that vitamin D plays a powerful role in preventing cancer and heart disease. But if you're like most Americans, chances are that you're on the low side for vitamin D because we don't spend enough time outdoors. In fact, at least half of all adults don't get enough. And according to a 2009 article in the medical journal *Pediatrics*, more than 6 million American kids—about one in five—are deficient in D.

VITAMIN D *with Frank Lipman, MD*

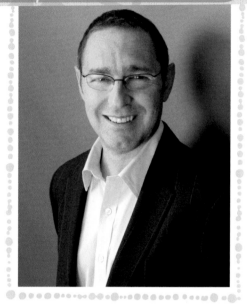

Although it's called a vitamin, vitamin D is more like a hormone, produced in the body, with far-reaching effects, influencing metabolic pathways, cellular functions, and the expression of myriad genes. By contrast, vitamins cannot be produced by your body. You get them from dietary sources.

Judging by what I see in my practice and speaking with colleagues around the world, we are facing a major vitamin D deficiency epidemic. It is now believed that vitamin D deficiency is the most common medical condition in the world, affecting over one billion people, with potentially grave consequences. It is a silent epidemic, because many people with low vitamin D levels remain asymptomatic.

Some of the more common symptoms of vitamin D deficiency are:

- Fatigue
- General muscle pain and weakness
- Tender sternum when you press on it
- Muscle cramps
- Joint pain
- Chronic pain
- Weight gain
- Restless sleep
- Poor concentration
- Headaches

Like all steroid hormones, vitamin D is involved in making hundreds of enzymes and proteins, which are crucial for preserving health and preventing disease. Virtually every tissue and cell in your body has a vitamin D receptor. Vitamin D has the ability to interact with and affect more than two thousand genes in the body. It enhances muscle strength, builds bone, has anti-inflammatory effects, and bolsters the immune system. It helps the action of insulin and has anti-cancer activity. Thus, vitamin D deficiency has been shown to play a role in almost every major disease, including:

- Osteoporosis (thin, brittle bones that break easily) and osteopenia (bones that are thinner than normal for your age)
- Seventeen varieties of cancer (including breast, prostate, and colon)
- Heart disease
- High blood pressure
- Obesity
- Metabolic syndrome (prediabetes) and diabetes
- Autoimmune diseases
- Multiple sclerosis

- Rheumatoid arthritis
- Infertility
- Depression
- Seasonal affective disorder
- Alzheimer's disease
- Fibromyalgia
- Chronic pain
- Psoriasis

The only test that can diagnose vitamin D deficiency is a 25-hydroxy-vitamin D (25 OH vitamin D) blood test. Unfortunately, some doctors order the wrong test, 1,25-dihydroxy-vitamin D. In fact, a common cause of high 1,25-dihydroxy-vitamin D is a low 25(OH)D or vitamin D deficiency. So when doctors see the 1,25-dihydroxy-vitamin D is normal or high, and tell their patients that they are okay, the patients are often vitamin D deficient. If you don't want to go through your doctor, ZRT Laboratory (zrtlab .com) offers a blood spot test that you can order.

Vitamin D is produced by your skin in response to exposure to ultraviolet radiation from the sun. In fact, this is such an efficient system that most of us make approximately 20,000 units of vitamin D after only twenty minutes of summer sun without suntan lotion (or clothes!). That's a hundred times more than the RDA! There must be a good reason why we make so much in so little time.

So why are we so scared to get some sun? For about the last twenty-five years, doctors (dermatologists in particular) have demonized sun exposure and repeatedly told us it is bad for us and causes cancer. But in the last few years, numerous studies have shown that modest exposure to sunlight helps the body produce the vitamin D it needs to keep bones healthy and protect against cancer, including skin cancer. Talk about a free natural treatment! Though

repeated sunburns—in children and very fair-skinned people—have been linked to melanoma, there is no credible scientific evidence that moderate sun exposure causes it. We evolved in the sun; we were made to get some sun, not to live our lives indoors and slather on sunscreen every time we go outside. Sunscreens, even weak ones, almost completely block your body's ability to generate vitamin D. Also, you don't generate vitamin D when sitting behind a glass window, whether in your car or at home, because the UV rays can't penetrate glass to generate vitamin D in your skin. As a general rule, if you aren't vitamin D–deficient, about twenty minutes a day of sun in the spring, summer, and fall on your face and arms or legs without sunscreen is adequate. It doesn't matter which part of the body you expose to the sun. Many people want to protect their face, so just don't put sunscreen on the other exposed parts for those twenty minutes.

If you live north of 37 degrees latitude (approximately a line drawn horizontally connecting Norfolk, Virginia, to San Francisco, California), sunlight is not sufficient to create vitamin D in your skin in the winter months, even if you are sitting in the sun in a bathing suit on a warm January day! The farther you live from the equator, the longer exposure you need to the sun in order to generate vitamin D.

You cannot get your requirements easily from your diet, because few foods naturally contain vitamin D. Some oily fish like wild salmon, mackerel, tuna and sardines, sun-dried shiitake mushrooms, and egg yolks are the best sources. Cod liver oil also contains vitamin D, as do fortified milk, orange juice, and cereal. But to get adequate amounts of vitamin D from food, you would have to eat two or three portions of wild salmon every day or drink twenty cups of fortified milk.

Besides the sun, the other reliable source of vitamin D is supplements, but taking the right amount is crucial. Most doctors tend to underdose. I prefer vitamin D_3. If you are vegan, you can use vitamin D_2 instead, which (unlike vitamin D_3) does not come from an animal source. However, it is not as biologically active or as effective as D_3.

How much vitamin D you need varies with age, body weight, percent of body fat, latitude, skin coloration, season of the year, use of sunblock, individual variation in sun exposure, and—probably—how ill you are. As a general rule, old people need more than young people, big people need more than little people, fat people need more than skinny people, dark-skinned people need more than fair-skinned people, northern people need more than southern people, winter people need more than summer people, sunblock lovers need more than sunblock haters, sun-phobes need more than sun worshipers, and ill people may need more than well people.

If your vitamin D blood level is above 45ng/ml and for maintenance, I recommend 2,000 to 4,000 IU daily, depending on the factors discussed above, if you know them. In other words if you are older, larger, living in the northern latitudes during the winter, are not getting sun, and have dark skin, I recommend the higher maintenance dose.

If your vitamin D blood level is 30 to 45 ng/ml, I recommend you correct it with 5,000 IU of vitamin D_3 a day for three months under a doctor's supervision and then recheck your blood levels.

If your blood level is less than 30 ng/ml, I recommend you correct it with 10,000 IU of vitamin D_3 a day under a doctor's supervision and then recheck your blood levels after three months. It usually takes a good six months to optimize your vitamin D levels if you're deficient. Once this occurs, you can lower the dose to the maintenance dose of 2,000 to 4,000 IU a day.

It is impossible to generate too much vitamin D in your body from sunlight exposure: Your body will self-regulate and only make what it needs. Although very rare, it is possible to overdose and become toxic with supplementation. Vitamin D is a fat-soluble vitamin and is therefore stored in the body for longer periods of time. If you're taking 5,000 IU or more daily, you should have your blood levels monitored approximately every three months.

Frank Lipman, MD, is the author of *Revive: Stop Feeling Spent and Start Living Again* and founder of the Eleven Eleven Wellness Center.

MULTI-SUPPLEMENTS

Aside from being careful to get enough vitamin B_{12} and vitamin D, you don't really have to worry about the other vitamins and minerals when you eat a mostly raw, vegan diet. Or do you? Stuff happens, and sometimes you can't eat the way you want to. And even when you can, other factors, like illness, food allergies, drug treatment, or even stress, mean that you might need extra on some vitamins and minerals.

To be on the safe side, I suggest taking a daily multivitamin/mineral supplement. Look for a brand that's designed for adults and has at least 100 percent of the RDA for vitamin B_{12} if you are not also taking any B_{12} or B complex supplements. Make sure that it's gluten-free and vegetarian. Quality counts in supplements—but that doesn't always translate into price. Expensive doesn't necessarily mean better. If you can't afford a pricey daily supplement, there are high-quality affordable brands of multivitamins on the market that make it possible for you to never skip a dose.

OMEGA-3 SUPPLEMENTS

As I explained in chapter 4, your body needs essential fatty acids such as omega-3s just as much as it needs vitamins. And just as I suggest taking vitamin supplements to be absolutely certain you're getting enough of what you need, I also suggest taking a daily omega-3 supplement. Look for one that gets the omega-3s from algae—that way you get a pure, animal-free product (no fish oil). I prefer enteric-coated capsules that don't dissolve until they enter your small intestine—this helps avoid stomach upset and burpiness.

Remember that the capsules are supplements, not substitutes. You still want to have plenty of natural omega-3 sources in your diet, including nuts, seeds, beans, and vegetable oils (especially flaxseed). How much should you take? Capsules range from 200 to 1,000 mg. Generally speaking 1,000 mg (1 gram) a day should be enough. Larger doses can thin your blood a bit, which might be bad for you.

A great vegetarian supplement to add to your wellness arsenal is a product called Life's DHA Omega 3 (learn more at lifesdha.com). Dr. Mehmet Oz first introduced me to this product when he made a house call to our Brooklyn pad to shoot my Oprah episode. The handsome and helpful doc arrived bearing gifts of a green drink, Life's DHA supplements, and a pair of scrubs (which I still write in—so comfy!).

DIGESTIVE ENZYMES

I suggest taking daily digestive enzyme supplements. They take some of the load off your digestive system and let your body divert that energy to other purposes. And they make sure you have the enzymes you need, when you need them, to digest your food thoroughly and get maximum nutrition from it.

Add a digestive enzyme to your diet, especially when you're eating animal products and/or cooked food. This will aid your body in proper digestion and elimination. Once we heat chow over 118 degrees, it loses its vitamins, minerals, and—most importantly—enzymes. Sooooo chow some enzymes to help everybody out!

You have a lot of choices when it comes to digestive enzymes—so many that this is one of the more confusing shelves at the health food store. Some supplements have ten or more enzymes in them. When making your choice, look for a supplement that has at least three kinds of enzymes: proteases, which help digest protein, amylases, which help digest carbohydrates, and lipases, which help digest fats. Some experts think you also need cellulase, an enzyme that helps break down insoluble fiber from cellulose, which is the main component of the cell walls in plants. Look for a supplement where the enzymes are all plant-based, since this is closer to what your body naturally produces. My favorites are sold at the Hippocrates Health Institute (hippocratesinst.org). They're called LifeGive HHI-Zymes, and they come in a bucket of 650 caps. Enzymetica brand (enzymedica.com) has several fantastic products. Whatever brand you go with, take one or two capsules with each meal.

ALOE VERA

Last but not least, I've been sucking on Aloe Life Herbal Aloe Detox Plus Formula (aloelife.com). I put a capful or two in a liter of water and drink it all morning. Aloe is more than just a great sunburn remedy. In fact, numerous studies have shown aloe vera to be a general boost for your overall immune system.

Research has shown three major areas where aloe is effective: anti-inflammatory, antibacterial, and antiviral. The juice is said to soothe digestive tract irritations such as colitis, ulcers, and irritable bowel syndrome, according to a paper in the *Journal of the American Osteopathic Society*.

In one study, asthmatic subjects took aloe orally for six months, and nearly half of them reported a reduction or elimination of asthma symptoms. Aloe also contains protein, calcium, magnesium, zinc, vitamins A, B_{12}, and E, and essential fatty acids; it's naturally rich in calcium, vitamin C, natural enzymes, and germanium, a mineral that may help people with immunodeficiency diseases, chronic pain, and heart and circulatory problems.

Natural anti-inflammatory substances and analgesics are present in the gel-like yellow sap of aloe's plump leaves, and that glorious goo can reduce swelling, pain, and skin irritation.

FULL SPECTRUM

For those of you who have never downed any kind of vitamin other than a chewable Fred Flintstone, the previous list might seem pretty long. Yet I've known people who take a separate carry-on when flying just to carry their vitamins, powders, potions, and pills! That's overdoing it. The CSD is super-healthy, and the aforementioned give your system an extra boost. My feeling is if you buy the best, most high-quality vegetarian supplements from reliable sources, they can play a part in your ongoing vitality, shimmer, and spark!

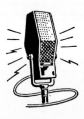

testimonial: Miri E.

I've been following Kris Carr and the Crazy Sexy lifestyle for about two years. I could go on and on about the physical benefits of this amazing lifestyle: clear skin, tons of energy and focus, my immune system is unbelievable, my blood tests are all fine, I'm strong and happy, and much more. For me, besides feeling incredible physically, the CSD minimized the monster in the big C and made it like a shadow on the wall. Kris Carr and the CSD lifestyle have given me what no one else could: empowerment! This lifestyle taught me how to live and be a better me. It shows me that I have choices and options; that I do not need to live with fear anymore. It taught me that I have a tremendous inner strength, and gave me lots of tools to live my life to the fullest. It taught me that canSer is not just about life and death, it's about doing and being my best in between; it taught me to be happy regardless. I learned that I can control what goes inside my body. I choose the best in every single bite and every single thought.

CHAPTER **9** IN REVIEW

REMEMBER:

- Food is the best source of nutrients, but we can also use a little help from our friends: supplements and superfoods.

- Probiotics are great for balancing good bacteria—look for one high in lactobacillus and bifidobacterium.

- Superfoods are rich in phytochemicals that reduce the risk of certain forms of cancer, reduce inflammation, strengthen the immune system, and in general contribute to a healthier, more fab you.

- Make sure you're getting enough B_{12}.

- Get your vitamin D from a supplement when you can't get it from the sun.

- Give your brain a boost with omegas.

- Digestive enzymes help what? Digestion!

- Aloe vera is anti-bad-stuff in a big way.

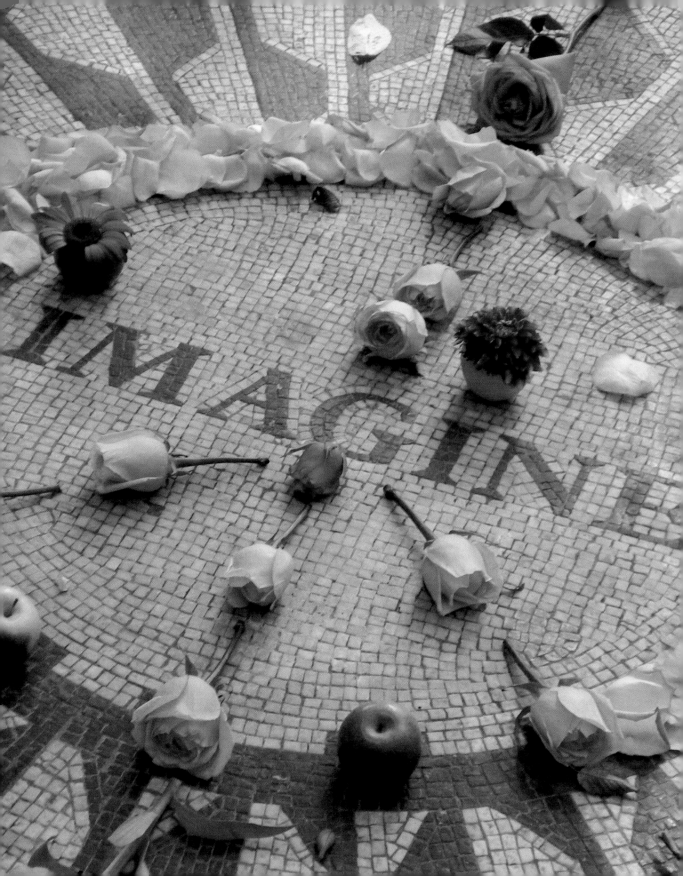

LET THE *adventure* CLEANSE BEGIN!

Your next great adventure—the 21-Day Cleanse—will tune your body, mind, and spirit. At the end of it, you'll feel magnificent and look beautiful inside and out. If you love the new you, keep going! The Crazy Sexy Diet is an optimum way of life. Let it be your foundation, a home base to come back to whenever you veer off. The cleanse is intended to give you freedom from obstruction and liberation from bullshit. It's not meant to create or support more stress in your life. As I said earlier, there's no such thing as perfection. Perfect is beige. Obsessing over every bite is completely contrary to the purpose and spirit of my book. Your overall goal is to have a peaceful feeling in your heart and

in your body. It's that simple. So don't be afraid, just get out there and do your thing! If you bottom out or revolt over the course of the 21 days, just giggle and recommit. Okay?

> **Your overall goal is to have a peaceful feeling in your heart and in your body.**

For the next three weeks, I offer daily inspiration, advice, and reminders. You'll find a week's worth of recipe suggestions starting on page 181. You'll notice that the daily entries look very different from many 7-, 14-, 21-, or 30-day "diet" plans you may have seen elsewhere. This is not a one-size-fits-all tune-up. There are no strict meal plans, measurements, calorie counting, minute-by-minute to-do lists, weigh-ins, or repetitive info. You're a big girl (or boy), and you're smarter (and busier) than that. Some days will naturally be more intense than others, so why force it? Besides, I've armed you with tons of info about eating, shopping, self-care, and other Crazy Sexy stuff. So you're coming into the cleanse with wisdom and confidence. Plus, I trust you.

What I will give you is far more powerful than serving size measurements. For the next 21 days, I'm going to help you change your mind, rebuild your self-esteem, and teach you how to smash fear in order to reach for your dreams. They're within your range ladies (and gents), you just have to stretch yourself and grab them.

To accomplish this, each day includes a focus, affirmation, prayer, diet or lifestyle tip, and God pod motivation to get your ass in gear. The prayers are in no way religious (unless you want them to be). They're more like mini conversations you have with yourself that remind you to honor the angel inside. Positive affirmations are the ultimate form of prayer: They rewire your subconscious mind and propel you toward the life you want.

Though I've mapped out the physical and emotional journey, you may experience symptoms, road bumps, and triumphs on different days. If so, just refer to the entry that suits you most. I also suggest you keep track of your progress in a journal that you keep alongside this book.

Remember, this isn't about deprivation! The Crazy Sexy Diet adds an abundance of healthy, spiritually wealthy food to your menu. Once you get over the initial detox hump and overcome

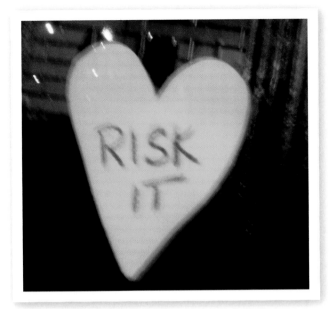

old cravings, you won't be hungry because you'll be eating the highest-quality nutrition on the planet. I know from experience you'll get into a groove and find the pattern that works for you while still following the basic guidelines.

If you need added help or a virtual shoulder to lean on, visit crazysexylife.com for mountains of support, community, cutting-edge articles, newsletters, and information about events, retreats, and online programs. Oh, and I hang out there, too, so if ya wanna gab, come find me. The wealth of information there is invaluable.

Now let's get started!

20 questions over 21 days

The following questions will help keep you on the right road over the next 21 days. Ideally you want to try to answer these questions at the end of the day when you can sit and think without distraction. Hey, why don't ya photocopy these pages to make up your own journal!

★ mark the circles for *yes!* or fill in the blank . . .

1   Did you abstain from coffee?

2   Did you abstain from alcohol?

3   Did you abstain from gluten?

4   Did you abstain from animal products?

5   Did you abstain from crack (aka sugar) and choose low-glycemic fruits and better alternatives such as stevia or agave?

6   Did you dry brush today?

7   Did you clean your sinuses with the good ol' neti pot?

8   Did you move your body for at least thirty-five minutes?

9   Did you meditate for fifteen to twenty minutes?

10 Did you chew your meals thoroughly and mindfully?

11 Did you laugh out loud and tell someone you loved him or her today?

12 Did you spend time in nature? Even five minutes is better than nothing.

13 Did you get eight hours of uninterrupted sleep?

14 What did you eat today and did you juice? Include breakfast, lunch, dinner, and any in-between snacking—it may help to jot down meals and snacks throughout the day.

15 How much purified water did you consume? You can include fresh veggie juices in your calculation.

16 What supplements did you take?

17 How was your elimination?

18 What time did you stop eating? Three hours before bed is optimum.

19 How do you feel physically?

20 How do you feel emotionally?

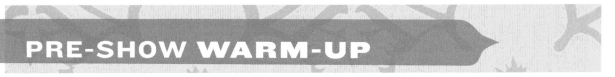

PRE-SHOW WARM-UP

It's best to transition for the week before you start. Consider it a wean week. After all, you're still a new colt learning to balance. No need to hit the racetrack day one. Choose a day to start and try not to begin during a time when you have lots of parties, weddings, birthdays, or the like. Though this is an easy way of life, you want to get the hang of it before prancing into an environment that's unsupportive of the new and improving you.

Get your cabinets, crisper, and appliances ready, line up your supplements, dust off your sneakers, make a massage appointment, buy an enema bag and research colon hydrotherapists in your area, get a fancy journal that inspires you, dig out a kitchen timer for your daily meditation practice, and review chapter 7 for other tips on God pod maintenance.

DURING WEAN WEEK:

- Slowly remove coffee if you haven't done so. Cut back to one cup per day and review my tips for transitioning in chapter 3.

- Cut back to no more than two alcoholic drinks per week and choose organic red wine.

- Hydration creates happy cells. Make sure you're drinking enough purified water. Stuff's gonna start to rumble—flush it out.

- Reduce your meat consumption to no more than 3 to 4 ounces twice a week.

- Phase out dairy and gluten. Include no more than two or three servings of each over the course of the week.

- Completely cut out processed sugar and refined carbs.

- Double up your intake of greens this week and dip your toe into the juicy world of juicing.

A crazy sexy DAY IN THE LIFE

A healthy, happy day rolls something like this . . . Pop open your peepers early. Brush your teeth, drink a large glass of purified water, and get your ass to the meditation cushion! Deal with your chaos for about fifteen to twenty minutes and follow it with green juice and other God pod maintenance (like dry brushing, neti, rebounding, yoga, etc.). Ideally you want to consume only liquids till noon. That means green juice, green smoothies, purified water, and teas. Keep in mind that you can have several servings. If that's not

enough for you, no worries, solid foods are definitely an option.

Lunch and dinner follow the 60/40 to 80/20 ratio. In simple speak: Slightly more than half of your plate should be covered with alkaline veggie dishes (salads, steamed or lightly sautéed greens and veggies). Got it? Take a look at the following menu sample for creative ideas. After that I leave the chow in your capable hands, and I'll deal with the emotional gunk! On the seventh day of each week, you will have the opportunity to fast—remember, this is optional. Review chapter 6 if you need a fasting refresher.

Here's how seven days might look for you. Again, this isn't a prescription, so you don't have to follow it to the letter. Remember that you can always amp up portion sizes when you like; the fun thing about this way of eating is that volume is okay! It just means more alkaline goodness. For some, this actually might seem like a lot of food! If you're used to a cup of coffee and a cracker, then heck yeah, feeding yourself an abundance of alkaline goodness might be hard at first. Listen to your body and adjust accordingly. As for dessert, I don't recommend planning on having it each night. But on nights when you really need a sweet treat, opt for 70 percent dark chocolate, a serving of seasonal fruit, or chocomole (see recipes in appendix).

HERE'S WHAT A *week* might look like:

MONDAY

Upon rising:
Warm water with lemon (optional pinch of cayenne)

Herbal tea

Breakfast:
Green juice, followed by fresh berries or 1 green apple

Lunch:
Tofu Eggless Salad

Gluten-free bread

Snack:
Apples, pears, or celery sticks with almond or cashew butter

Dinner:
Thai "Peanut" Sauce Vegetables with quinoa

Shaved Kale Avocado Salad

TUESDAY

Upon rising:
Warm water with lemon (optional pinch of cayenne)

Herbal tea

Breakfast:
Green Guru Smoothie

Lunch:
Mexican Pilaf

Large salad with tons of goodies and your choice of dressing

Snack:
Hummus with gluten-free crackers

Dinner:
Teriyaki Tofu

Cabbage Hemp Salad

WEDNESDAY

Upon rising:
Warm water with lemon (optional pinch of cayenne)

Herbal tea

Breakfast:
Green juice till noon

Vanilla Chia Tapioca Pudding if you need more fuel

Lunch:
I Am Loved Nori Rolls

Ginger-Lemongrass Miso Soup

Snack:
Green juice

10–15 raw almonds

Dinner:
Roasted Tomatoes Stuffed with Pine Nut Spinach Pâté and Young Dill

Mediterranean Quinoa Salad with Capers

THURSDAY

Upon rising:

Warm water with lemon (optional pinch of cayenne)

Herbal tea

Breakfast:

Apple Sprout Smoothie

Optional sprouted grain cereal with nut milk or seed milk (you can purchase these)

Lunch:

Tomato Wild Rice Soup

Simple Mediterranean Salad with Caper Berries

Snack:

Green juice

10–15 raw almonds

Dinner:

Buddha Bowl

Marinated Sea Vegetables

Miso Broth with Zucchini Somen and Shiitake

FRIDAY

Upon rising:

Warm water with lemon (optional pinch of cayenne)

Herbal tea

Breakfast:

Urban Zen Juice till noon

Gluten-free toast with avocado and sea salt (if desired)

Lunch:

Olive Quesadillas

Large salad with tons of goodies and your choice of dressing

Snack:

Veggie crudités with hummus, bean dip, or dressing

Dinner:

Woodstock Peace Salad with choice of dressing

Southwest Black Bean and Roasted Sweet Potato Burger

SATURDAY

Upon rising:

Warm water with lemon (optional pinch of cayenne)

Herbal tea

Breakfast:

Green juice till noon

Sexy Seed Cakes (if needed)

Lunch:

Choosing Raw "Peanut" Noodles with steamed veggies (sprinkle with sea salt, Bragg's apple cider, or oil and lemon)

Snack:

Green juice

1–2 rice cakes with raw almond butter

Dinner:

Asian Medley

Palak Paneer

SUNDAY

Happy fasting day! See chapter 6 for a refresher.

Check out the Raw Goddess Soup in the recipe section.

Got it? Ok, now let's get started on the next 21 days!

the
**21-DAY
CLEANSE**

Day 1
21-DAY CLEANSE

Ta da! It's Day 1 of the Tune-up. Your big task this week is to balance between pushing yourself out of your comfort zone and being gentle with yourself. There's no need to be in it to "win" it. Be in it to do better, feel better, to stretch your self-imposed limitations—that's more than enough.

Today you will remove coffee completely. Yup, give it up. If you are still consuming animal flesh and dairy, say so long. Since tush is a thing of the past (or at least it is for the next 21 days) it's time to add a vitamin B_{12} and B complex supplement to your diet. Gluten is out. The only way you'll know if you are sensitive is to boot it for now. Refined sugars and processed carbs are way out. See ya!

FOCUS

What you focus on for the next 21 days is extremely important. I want you to concentrate on the positive rather than the negative. Instead of "I didn't do it right," I want you to think of all that you did accomplish. To do this, you really need to think about the language you use. We all talk to ourselves. Take stock of what you are saying and remember that your cells have ears! They're listening.

PRAYER

Please help me open my mind. Ignite my childlike curiosity and anything-is-possible attitude. Tap me on the shoulder if I act like a cranky old bat. The voices that hold me back are thoroughly misinformed. Grant me the wisdom to release them now.

AFFIRMATION

I am capable, confident, intelligent, resilient and in charge. Health and happiness are my birthrights and I accept with gratitude.

BREAKFAST

Drink a large glass of purified water with lemon, and add a wee dash of cayenne to awaken your circulation; followed by herbal tea, one to two cups of green or white tea, or yerba mate. When you're hungry, sip 16 ounces of fresh organic green juice or green smoothie (see the recipe section for examples). If you're still hungry have more juice and/or smoothie.

LUNCH

Load 60 to 80 percent of your plate with a rainbow colored salad, good fats, and other raw delights. Yummy "peanut" noodles, raw veggie pasta, nut pâté, and jicama nori rolls are lovely choices. You may not need more. However, the remaining 20 to 40 percent of your plate can be graced with healthy and whole cooked fare (slightly steamed or sautéed veggies, beans, tempeh, tofu, gluten-free grains and pastas, soup, baked sweet potato or nori rolls, etc.). Review the sample recipe section and reading list for more ideas—and crazysexylife.com has hundreds more recipes waiting for you to explore!

SNACK

The juice bar is open and it's cocktail hour! Around 3 to 4 p.m. we all crash. Instead of grabbing adrenal smacking stimulants, the new you will guzzle a large and perky green juice! If you want more, go for a handful of raw almonds or brown rice cakes with hummus, or tahini or guacamole, flax crackers, bean dip, and so on. Get creative!

If you're a girl or guy on the go, bring snacks with you. That way you won't be tempted to swerve into a mini mart or vending machine. A small travel cooler with ice packs will help keep juice and other perishables fresh. Many stevia brands come in handy packets for your purse, so stock up. Raw nuts and seeds are also great for your desk drawer. Just don't overdo it—these are really nutritious and a great source of good fats, but the calories can add up.

DINNER

Same ratios as lunch—so simple you don't even have to think about it. An average night at chez Carr/Fassett is super easy. We make a lovely salad with romaine, tomatoes, snap peas, hemp seeds, red onions, oil-cured olives, and an easy agave mustard dressing. For the cooked portion, we make a Buddha Bowl with quinoa, broccoli, chick peas, garlic, Braggs liquid, black pepper, cayenne, and some flax oil. I serve myself a huge portion of salad (60-80 percent of my plate) and a smaller portion of the Buddha bowl (20-40 percent of my plate).

DESSERT

Huh? Well, if ya need it and you don't have a major health issue or a sweet tooth that transforms you into a werewolf, a little dark chocolate (at least 70%), cacao pudding, or a square of carob from time to time won't kill ya. I make my own chocolate with 100% cacao and stevia or yacon. Please note that dessert on a regular basis will slow down the cleanse process. But if you're going to snap without a treat, then snap off a piece of yummy, and STAY ON TRACK!

GOD POD MAINTENANCE

MOOOOVE! Sweat your prayers, walk, run, dance, play with Fido—whatever yanks your crank. I urge you to do 35 minutes a day at least five days a week. In addition, make sure to dry brush before you shower. Start at your toes and work up to your nose! If you can do regular saunas, or, even better, infrared saunas, during this time, ooh la la—speed the success!

TIP

Optimally you want to drink green juice or green smoothies until noon and then add solids at lunch and dinner. However, if you still feel hungry after a couple of juices, wait 20 minutes, and then enjoy a bowl of low-glycemic berries. When consuming fruit, please eat it alone. Other breakfast options include gluten-free toast with Earth Balance or avocado with a dash of sea salt, almond butter with celery, raw cereals or gluten-free cooked cereals, oatmeal, seed pancakes, nut milk, chia pudding, and of course there's always the leftover veggies and grains from the night before! Finally, remember to CHEW! Can you try 20 chews per bite? If so—wow, will your tummy and tubes love you.

Day 2
21-DAY CLEANSE

You did it! Day 1 is over and you are one step closer to liberation. What you leave out of your diet is as important as what you include. The healthiest diets have one thing in common: They toss crappy food. This diet and lifestyle is the Rolls-Royce, and you deserve an elegant ride.

FOCUS

Embrace yourself—literally. You may feel tired and cranky today. Yesterday you started what is a major shift in your life and health—but it likely brought up all sorts of physical and emotional pangs. That's okay! Stop what you are doing right now (well, after you read my directions), take in a very deep breath, and raise your hands to the heavens. Let your capable hands meet in a prayer. Stretch your God pod and while you swoop your lovely arms down exhale all the air out and hug yourself. As you embrace your majesty, say this out loud: "I LOVE YOU (fill in your name)." Repeat three times.

PRAYER

May I know in my heart that I am precious, worthy, and divine (aka very fabulous!). When I move from my own private divinity, whatever I do is enough.

AFFIRMATION

I *love* my thighs. My skin is *beautiful*. My organs are healthy and powerful.

GOD POD MAINTENANCE

It doesn't matter what time of day you do it—just do it! Exercise for thirty-five minutes. There is no way out of this, so don't try to wiggle. Oh, and how's the meditation going, dear one? Don't blow it off, okay? Who cares if your mind stages a mutiny? What matters is that you show up.

TIP

Plan meals ahead of time. It's a huge help! Though I'm not going to tell you what to eat every step of the way, that doesn't mean you shouldn't strategize. Don't get caught with your dinner pants down, sister. Crack open your cookbooks, shop, and plot. Stack the odds for success in your favor.

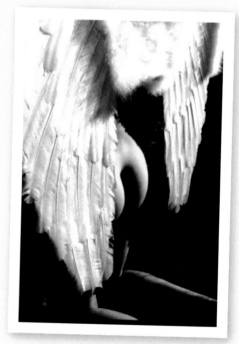

Wednesday—hump day. You may hit your first real wall today. Brava! Hit it and then climb it, champ. It's really just a speed bump. You may feel some physical detox symptoms, such as fatigue, headache, a foggy brain, skin rashes, and muscle weakness. That's okay; it's normal. Your body will jump at the opportunity to remove stored toxins. This is training wheels week, so stay where you are and grin and bear it.

FOCUS

In your mind's eye, imagine how good it feels to start something new and see it to completion. For a minute or two, close your eyes and picture a colorful calendar. Watch yourself as you check off each day of the cleanse with a green marker. Let the joy wash over you as you usher your accomplishment into your tissues. You did it! Now open your eyes and know that you will do it, to the best of your ability at this time. The only failure is inaction.

PRAYER

Allow me to let go of the restraints and get out of my own way. I am as free as I will let myself be, and I could really use a gentle reminder (and perhaps a flick on the ass).

AFFIRMATION

I am so frickin' cool and delicious and pretty and witty and sharp! I love every inch of me! Who wouldn't?

GOD POD MAINTENANCE

Work it, girl, work it! Your lymph needs you. Hey, cutie, this is also a great day to play with your neti pot. Your sinuses and lungs will bow to you.

TIP

If you're jonesing for a frappuccino or Cinnabon, refer to tips for cutting cravings down to size in chapter 3.

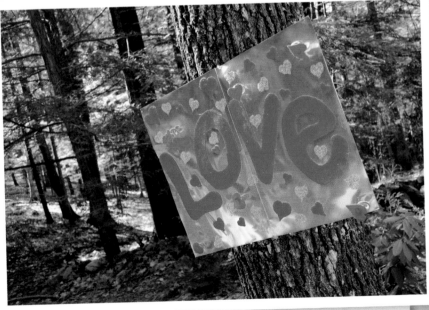

Remember when we were kids and we imagined we'd have our very own amusement park, along with two pet dinosaurs and a rocket for getting to school? Not only did we think it, we believed it to our core. Then one day a ninny of a neighbor pierced the dream with really dumb words: "Suzie, you can't own a rocket or a dinosaur. That's just silly." Your response: "What?" Followed by tears, snot, and disillusionment. Likewise, the new you may scare people because it forces them to look in the mirror. You may start hearing the voice of negativity from friends, family, and acquaintances starting about now and continuing in the future. Don't let the judgment of others who are less supportive of or puzzled (and maybe threatened) by your new lifestyle bring you down.

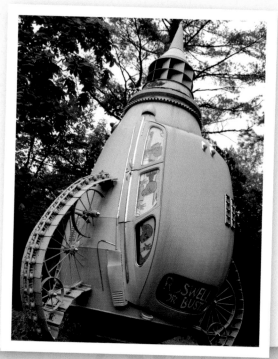

Understand that they just don't understand. Reassure them that you're happy and getting healthier. Do it nicely, with love.

FOCUS

Let your goals, no matter how big, be and feel real to you. Suck them in, smell and lick them. You have nothing to lose! Oh, and release the ninny. You may still be holding on to her words even though she's long gone from your life.

PRAYER

Please help me locate my inner rebel. May I become a trailblazing leader, not a follower. When I stand in my fully actualized glory, I encourage others to do the same.

AFFIRMATION

I have unlimited health, spiritual wealth, and happiness now. I am precious and I have so much to offer. The world needs me today.

GOD POD MAINTENANCE

You have an ass, so shake it. How many minutes can you spare? Let's try thirty-five! Hula would be very fun, don't you agree? Notice your breath as you exercise. Are you holding it or breathing too shallow? Combining deep breathing with exercise stimulates your lymph system and helps move toxins out of your body. Now that you adore your neti pot, you probably love the sinus ease it creates! Breathe, baby, breathe!

TIP

Snack on sunshine. That's right! Smokers take cig breaks and that seems to be perfectly acceptable. Why can't you take a twenty-minute sun break for some free vitamin D?

You might hit the TGIF terrors today. Friday can be scary for those of you who have traditionally designated it as the start of two days of indulgence, drinking, and sleeping in. Some strategic planning on how you'll handle festivities with friends that in the past led to eating crap, drinking poison, and general debauchery is in order. Celebrate your spirit without booze-filled spirits. Vodka tonics and limes will always be there. For now, just stick with the lime.

FOCUS

If you think you might slip over the weekend, plan your response now. This way when the urge rears its savage head, you'll be ready. When the going gets tough, the tough get grounded! Take a moment to feel your feet on the floor, be aware of your butt cheeks on the chair, take a few deep breaths, and let the temptation pass. Ask yourself what you really want. Chances are it has nothing to do with food. Maybe you need a hug or a nap or a talk with a trusted therapist. If you have to have this chat with yourself on the can in a public bathroom—so be it. Worse things have happened on that can!

PRAYER

May I share my shine without dimming it. Help me socialize with integrity. By setting an example, I inspire others. Remind me when I forget and fill me with holy shazzam discipline.

AFFIRMATION

When I put my mind to it, I can do anything. I am Wonder Woman and I wear bulletproof cuffs. I am able to wrangle my cravings with my Magic Lasso and remove them via my Invisible Plane—I'm in charge!

GOD POD MAINTENANCE

Meditation doesn't mean relaxation. Meditation is work and I sure hope you're doing it! If it was good enough for the Beatles, it's good enough for you! They meditated twenty minutes every day, and those dudes turned out pretty good.

TIP

Dine with the divine . . . Try to finish your meal three hours before bed. Your body repairs at night. Don't add to the burden by making it digest as well.

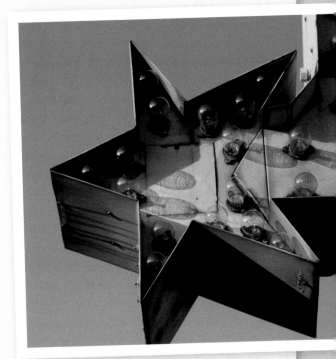

Day 6
21-DAY CLEANSE

Emotional detox symptoms are very, very normal. Irritability and feeling a little depressed and teary is part of the process (especially if you happen to have your period). You've removed the food vices that covered your pain, the snacks that created a false sense of joy (for like thirty seconds). Good for you! Substances that make us numb out are veils. Wear them on your wedding if you want, but not for the rest of your life. I promise the clouds will clear very soon—but they will come back if you don't do some emotional weeding.

FOCUS

You! Put some time aside to rest and refresh today. Take stock of your week and please write in your journal about your challenges, your victories, and any tips that can help you in the weeks to come. Make sure to use kind language. When you're done scribbling, go do something lovely for lovely you. Mani? Rub? Walk? Tea with a fun friend? Free time spent without food might leave you feeling, well, aimless. Fill it with experiences that can become wonderful memories. At the end of our lives, memories are all we have. Make lots of them!

PRAYER

May I be happy and free. May I be loving and loved. May I be healthy and whole.

AFFIRMATION

Each step is a victory. Each fall is a lesson. Either way, I am improving now.

GOD POD MAINTENANCE

Add in a few long, luxurious stretches after your exercise routine. Include affirmations with every move. Touch your toes: I am flexible. Twist to the side: I am gutsy. Reach for the sky: I am expansive. Bend over backward: I am lean. Stand on your head: I am a great chef!

TIP

Shop. For spinach, not shoes. You have another big week ahead, and tomorrow is a fasting day—prep for it sassy. Also, make sure you are drinking enough water, getting enough of the good fats, and chomping your greens. You shouldn't be hungry. Yes, you may be losing weight, but that's a side effect, not the main point. If you're a normal weight or on the thin side and feel you're losing too many pounds, add more nuts and seeds (whole or as butters), cooked grain, gluten-free bread, and other higher-calorie foods like avocados. If you're overweight, the CSD will bring your body into balance naturally.

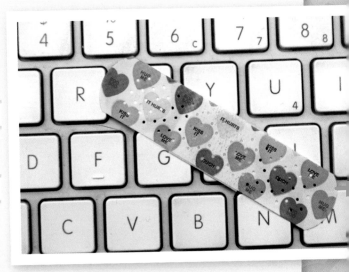

You may be fasting for part of the day today or for all of it. Do what feels right for you and listen to your body. Whatever you decide, keep hydrated and juicy.

FOCUS

Techno detox! Yesterday you cleansed emotions; today you'll cleanse the need to obsessively check your inbox. As Timothy Leary said, "Tune in, turn on, drop out"—of technology! That's right, fast from pixels. When you realize you're spending more time Googling fun stuff than actually doing it, you have to replace online noodling with real-world alternatives. Too much time sitting and surfing creates back problems, dry eyes, carpal tunnel, sleep issues, and even migraines. Change your relationship to technology. Start by meditating on ways you can structure your techno time better. Consider these:

- Pick up the phone old-school style, rather than shooting out endless e-mails.
- Check your e-mail only at scheduled times— 10 a.m., 2 p.m., 4 p.m.—and turn off the sound notification while you're at it.
- Limit online multitasking. You get less done than you think when you do this.
- Cease and desist on the Facebook ex-boyfriend snoop.
- Use an e-mail auto responder when you need to get caught up or just want a time-out. I used an auto responder, for the last six months of writing this book, and I couldn't have finished it without it. Here's what I wrote . . .

Cherished friends,

I am on a tight writing deadline for my next book. As a result, I may not be able to get back to you anytime soon. If this is urgent, please contact my assistant.

Peace, love, and veggies,

Kris Carr

- If you tweet, do it with purpose and not during dinner. No one really cares that you just wiped your ass. Twitter is for brand building, not senseless narcissistic drivel.

PRAYER

In this chaotic world, help me find peace, and remind me to limit the distractions that keep me from embracing my self-care. Impossible deadlines and stress create acidity in my body. The world won't blow up if I take a day off.

AFFIRMATION

I am calm and light. I am peaceful and easygoing. I find beauty in simplicity.

GOD POD MAINTENANCE

Get your cute ass outside in nature. Go to the beach, hit a mountain trail or local park, climb a tree, hunt waterfalls. I don't care if it's only 10 degrees outside and you'd rather cuddle with your laptop. Don't. Wrap yourself up like a warm burrito and let the cold wind slap you silly. Follow with a hot shower and essential oils skin elixir. Mix 15 to 20 drops of your fave essential oil with a jojoba, avocado, coconut, or sweet almond "carrier" oil for a healthy all-over moisturizer.

TIP

Kill your television! No Internet tonight, either. I betcha there's a great book on your shelf that would really love to be held. Books have feelings, too!

You did it! Week 1 is under your belt and no matter how it went, the hardest part is behind you. There will be more icy patches ahead (detox symptoms can pop up at any time), but you've taken some heroic steps. I wish you could see me giving you a standing ovation!

FOCUS

Everything you need to learn in life, you can learn from a chair. The diet is the seat (the largest area of focus); the mind, body, spirit, and daily practice are the four legs. When any one is off, we topple. Which one is off, doll? Pick one area of focus this week and crank it up!

PRAYER

My body is a blessing. I am so grateful to live in this beautiful temple. Please show me corners I didn't know existed. Please help me tend to those corners.

AFFIRMATION

I am graceful. I am fierce. I am gentle. I am a powerhouse. I am silly. I am serious. I love all my opposites and I am balancing them with ease.

GOD POD MAINTENANCE

Pump iron! Every pound of muscle in your body burns about 35 to 50 calories a day, while a pound of fat burns only around 2 calories. Strength training literally keeps your metabolism firing. Experts suggest thirty minutes of strength training two to three times a week. Exercise bands are another way to build strength. The bands are pretty and portable. Shove them in your purse and hit the park! Because you fasted yesterday, you may want to give yourself an enema followed by some probiotics today or get a colonic for a deeper cleaning. Fasting rustles up the gunk. Help move it out!

TIP

Have compassion. Sometimes it's hard to show yourself compassion. If that's the case, do it for the animals, the planet, the big picture. I protest suffering by voting with my fork and spending my dollars where they matter. Or better yet, do it for your children. Let the legacy of deprivation end with you.

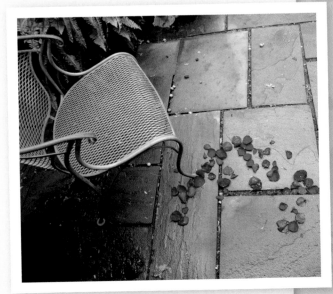

How's your belly treating you, love? You may be a little constipated, or perhaps you're experiencing the opposite—what my mom calls "the scoots." Either way, it's pretty normal. You're cleansing and rebuilding while flooding and flushing. The payoff comes with consistency. Fiber is like dumbbells for your tubes, making them stronger. Perhaps you're eliminating like a champ (one to three times per day) and you wonder if that's natural. Yes! If you're visiting the loo more than usual, rejoice. If not, check out products like Oxy-Mag or Natural Calm and a good probiotic. You may need a little help to get things moving.

FOCUS

Notice your bowels today. Ladies were taught not to poop or puff. Undo that ridiculous domestication. Gas is good. Poop is great. Tight jeans are silly. Let your belly breathe.

PRAYER

Sometimes I'm really uptight and impatient. Please help me turn my pounding fists into open receiving hands.

AFFIRMATION

I let go with ease. I am a clear channel. Energy flows through me, and all good things come to me.

GOD POD MAINTENANCE

Speaking of constipation, chemical-laden deodorants constipate your armpits. Check out skindeep.org for deodorant suggestions. Hugo Naturals Sea Fennel & Passionflower is my personal fave.

TIP

If you're experiencing gas or bloating, try to be more consistent about food combining. Take a digestive enzyme with your meals and don't drink water while you eat.

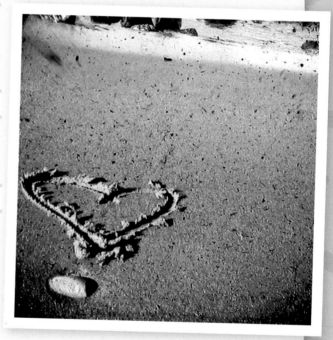

You've made it to double digits! Hip hip hooray! So how ya feeling, Wellness Warrior? We're powering our bodies with nature's electricity in order to shoot to the beautiful stars. But that doesn't mean we always feel good while on the trip. No doubt you felt some emotional and physical roller coasters last week. This week you might be really pissed off at me, the book, the cleanse, the world, yourself, the mailman, the president, everyone. It's just withdrawal symptoms, but it does not mean your feelings aren't valid and important. Notice and acknowledge them. But don't let 'em tell you what to do. What's really behind the tantrums? Are you having difficulty installing healthy boundaries? Saying no is a very liberating experience! If we say yes when we mean no, emotional chaos follows. If you're hitting some hot pockets, let yourself vent it out. Get ye to thy journal, unbridled wench! Get thyself to the mountain top and scream thy head off!

FOCUS

Meet your priestess. She is a force of nature. She adores sex, sauntering in red heels, free speech, and loud laughter. The priestess is deeply loving and compassionate but she'll fight to the death to protect her inner kid. Oh, and she smells good, too—like patchouli and rose with a splash of Egyptian musk. If your priestess has been amputated in any way, heal her.

PRAYER

Knowing I am loved and beautiful inside and out, may I embrace my feminine energy. Guide me back to my priestess and teach me never to leave her again.

AFFIRMATION

I am ripe with power, passion, and sizzle. I love and cherish my femininity.

GOD POD MAINTENANCE

Dance naked. Follow it up with a candlelit, hot soak. A couple of drops of rosemary, lavender, or pine essential oil relax the muscles and the mind. Sit back and sip some herbal tea while you're at it.

TIP

Include some "functional food" in your salad today. Kimchi or other naturally fermented veggies (available in the refrigerated section of natural and organic food stores) do wonders for your friendly flora.

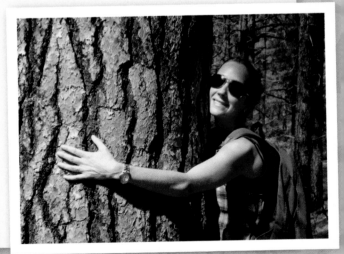

Yesterday you set about acknowledging your frustrations and anger. Today, start paying attention to those moments when you feel—out of the blue—fabulous. Many people experience a sense of well-being and even euphoria in the middle of a cleanse. You're eating a lot of mood foods—stuff that's better than Prozac with fewer side effects. Love these feelings and they'll love you back by multiplying. Love yourself and the world around you and you'll experience heaven on earth. If you have a hard time pinpointing what you love, maybe you're just out of practice. I'll help you jog your memory!

FOCUS

Make a love list—ten things you absolutely love. Love is a magnetic force that attracts an infinite amount of goodness into our cells. Love makes us radiant. Notice the love and invite it to tea. Give your darlings validation no matter how small or seemingly insignificant. This simple act reminds us that life is full of blessings. It's amazing how many beautiful things we notice when we train our eyes.

PRAYER

Allow me to notice the miracles and majesty in my life—noticing the magic helps me notice myself.

AFFIRMATION

I love how wonderful I feel and I am so incredibly proud of myself, right now, today.

GOD POD MAINTENANCE

If it's nice out, take a bike ride. If it's crappy outside (or cold) crank up the heat to 75 for thirty minutes and have a warm yoga session. Next, book a massage and write it in red ink on your calendar.

TIP

Sprout! Mung bean sprouts are an incredibly nutritious addition to your salad. You can find exact sprouting directions at sproutman.com. Here's my down-and-dirty version: Soak the beans in warm water overnight. Drain them in a colander and rinse several times over the course of a day or so. When their little tails grow to about an inch (give or take), they're ready to chow. Store them in the refrigerator.

I love . . . ♡

Pens with purple ink

Snuggling with my dog Lola

Claw-foot tubs and chandeliers

Bob Dylan

Cheating at Boggle

Sweatpants

Rhinestone hair clips

Greg Smithey from the Buns of Steel workout video (my mom loves him, too)

Doodling in the columns of official documents

When my handsome husband cleans the juicer

Day 12
21-DAY CLEANSE

Gratitude is the attitude!

Now that you've identified what you love, it's a delicious time to welcome gratitude into your life. Gratitude puts you in a position of having instead of wanting. When I take stock of my blessings, I get more blessings. When I throw bottomless "wanting" out into the universe, I get back more wanting. Life doesn't start when all your ducks are in a row; it's happening right now. Notice what you do have instead of focusing on what you don't. Plenty multiplies like horny bunnies, but so does lack. If you can't think of anything, then your inner sourpuss has hijacked you. This is very serious. Immediately send a SWAT team armed with a fire hose of sunshine to your rescue.

FOCUS

Here's something for you to mull over. What if your problems disappeared today? Would you be instantly happy? Tell the truth. My sense is that the answer would be no. Most of us build state-of-the-art infrastructure to house our ego's negative voice. We provide sturdy platforms for doubt and despair. If the source of the misery were removed, don't think for a nanosecond that the self-created support beams would vanish with it. When you stop feeding the negativity, it will collapse.

PRAYER

With gratitude for all that I have, remind me to take stock and be thankful for another day on Mama Earth.

AFFIRMATION

My life is abundant now; rivers of joy and health flood my inner ashram and fill me with stamina, strength, and amen.

GOD POD MAINTENANCE

Download a guided meditation or peaceful chanting CD. Take fifteen minutes or more to rest and regroup.

TIP

Clean out the makeup bag and medicine cabinet. Be grateful that you have alternatives—and use them. Chemical moisturizers, old lipsticks and eye shadows—gotta go.

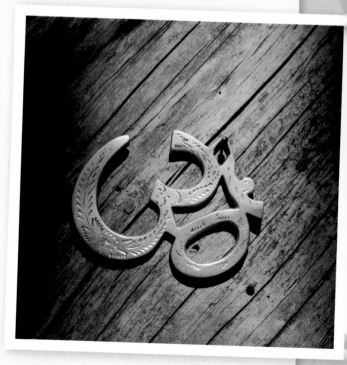

Making meals for yourselves and others is a profound way to share love. As you get more comfortable with your ability to make tasty cuisine, invite folks over to break (gluten-free) bread. Just because you're cleansing doesn't mean you have to isolate. Share your knowledge. The world needs you! Teach your coworkers how to juice. Make a healthy lunch for your mom and share the recipe. You're the sexiest Prevention Is Hot cheerleader I have ever seen—shake those pom-poms!

FOCUS

Be the change you wish to see in the world. (That's not my genius—that's Gandhi. He's hot.)

PRAYER

Allow me to help others find their core vitality. Help me to share my knowledge in a way that people can understand. Though I am excited, I realize that people don't like being bashed over the head. Help me teach with patience and compassion.

AFFIRMATION

I have the amazing ability to clearly communicate my wisdom to others.

GOD POD MAINTENANCE

Tongue scraping, anyone? Ever notice the whitish coating that sometimes collects on your tongue? That's waste products and bacteria. Help your tongue out by gently removing it. You can find a scraper at any health food or drugstore—they cost about $2. French kissing is a lot better with a clean tongue!

TIP

When making meals for meat-loving carnivores, choose a hearty, well-seasoned dish that will wow them—roasted veggies, a raw lasagna, tempeh Reuben, or rich grain dishes and soups. Then how about a lush dessert? Kick off the festivities with fresh juice served in a sexy wine goblet or champagne flute.

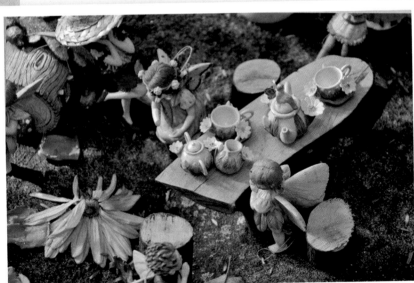

Day 14
21-DAY CLEANSE

Guess what? It's fasting day again. If you're up for it, fantastic! If not, just eat light and bright today. One of the benefits of fasting is mental clarity and spiritual purification. Fasting gets rid of excess. It peels off the layers of dullness revealing a holy honey core. Some of the greatest spiritual teachers, activists, artists, and philosophers used periodic fasts to connect with a deeper layer of self. Gandhi, Buddha, Jesus, Mother Teresa, Plato, Aristotle, Abraham Lincoln, and Leonardo da Vinci are among some of the fasting hall of famers. Buddha's experience with fasting is très Crazy Sexy. While he did experiment with longer fasts, Buddha found them too extreme (me too!). Instead he opted for the one-day tune-up that led him to the middle way and enlightenment. Buddha is hot!

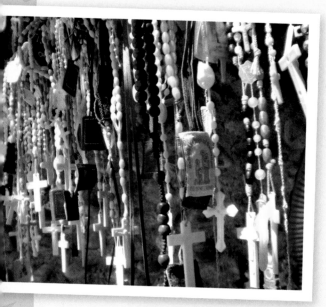

FOCUS

Think about other areas of excess in your life. Closets? File cabinets? How about your Rolodex? Whoa. This may be time for a little house-cleaning, and not just with the mop and broom. It's time to detox the little black book. You just don't have enough energy to tap yourself out with people who take, take, take. The people who really matter will step up to the plate.

PRAYER

With a loving heart, help me to release the relationships that bring me down. I bless them and send them to the light so I don't have to haul their tired asses around in my mind. Guide me to surround myself with people who give and receive with ease.

AFFIRMATION

I am a magnet of goodness and starlight. Like attracts like. The relationships in my life are nurturing and I am supported today.

GOD POD MAINTENANCE

Review the section on Reiki in chapter 7 and give yourself some healing energy. Take a salt or cider bath after your thirty-five-minute move-and-shake session.

TIP

How are those catnaps coming? Are you training yourself to shut down and tune out? Oh, and are you getting eight hours of nightly snooze?

Let's be real. Sometimes forgiveness can feel like a four-letter cuss word. We all have a hard time letting go of people, memories, and situations that hurt us. But holding on to grudges keeps us prisoner. Wanna liberate? Choose peace. It's a one-way ticket to wellness. This doesn't mean you have to invite your enemy to dinner and hug or that you should dismiss abuse or neglect. It means that your health is your first priority and anything that blocks the flow has got to go! Release the negative emotions that fester and lower your vitality. Forgive.

Sometimes the hardest thing to forgive is your body. Perhaps you feel that it has betrayed you in some way. Try to reframe the issue. If it were a professor, what would it be trying to teach you? Become aware of the lesson.

If you can, forgive your family, friends, enemies, cells, bones, tissues, and most importantly, yourself.

FOCUS

Write a list of people, situations, and body parts that you need to forgive.

PRAYER

Help me to let go of the pain and forgive.

AFFIRMATION

Through the power of forgiveness all emotional and physical obstacles melt away. I embrace my past and look forward to my future. Today, I forgive.

GOD POD MAINTENANCE

Take fun seriously. Plan for it. Put it on the calendar. Fun is nonnegotiable, and fun helps you

to do what? Forgive! Try rebounding. Jumping on a mini-trampoline burns about 100 calories in fifteen minutes. That's nothing to sneeze at. Trampoline playtime moves trapped fat out of tissues, cells, and thighs. Blast your favorite tunes and bounce to the sky. If you can't invest in a tramp at this time, buy a jump rope and "Skip to My Lou, my darlin'."

TIP

Make your own trail mix. Dried fruits like goji berries are low glycemic, and because they have the same transit time they combine well with nuts. Try goji, raw macadamias or cashews, mulberries, and some raw cacao nibs. Call it Forgiveness Trail Mix and enjoy some while blessing the experiences that make you the strong person you are today.

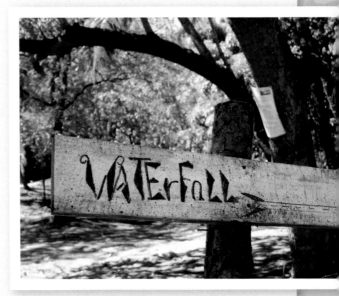

Part of what you might need to shake your groove thing and live like you mean it is to travel. No fear. You can go all over tarnation with the Crazy Sexy lifestyle.

FOCUS

Adventure! You're not living on an island (unless of course, you live on an island). Nothing can stop you from sightseeing in your own backyard, across town, or across the globe.

PRAYER

Grant me the wisdom to see beyond my boundaries.

AFFIRMATION

I am a global God(dess), open to the world.

GOD POD MAINTENANCE

Dry brush? Check. Thirty-five-minute jog, walk, tumble, roll, or bounce? Check. Neti pot? Check. How about getting your eyebrows shaped by a follicle master? Your brows are the frames that highlight your beauty. Tend to them.

TIP

Read my friend Emily Deschanel's advice about eating Crazy Sexy on the road.

GO VEGAN *with Emily Deschanel*

It hasn't always been easy being green— or vegan. I'm an actor, so I often find myself on location or in circumstances that don't lend themselves easily to healthy eating. Traveling and location work requires a little extra planning.

Always do Internet research before you go anywhere. Print out a list of health food stores, farmers' markets, and restaurants in the area where you are visiting. I also look up juice bars before leaving for a trip. Juice makes me feel better and healthier, and brings my body back to normal after being messed up by flying. Happy cow.net is one Web site that helps you find restaurants with vegetarian or veggie-friendly food and health food stores across the country.

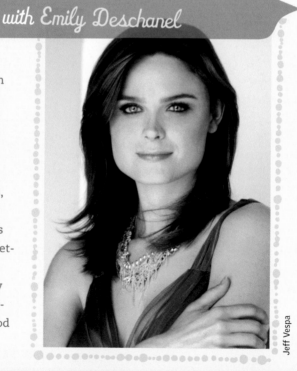
Jeff Vespa

Healthy Highways (healthyhighways.com) is an excellent guidebook for healthy eating across the country. Many mobile phones have applications that help traveling vegetarians, too; http://groovyvegetarian.com/2009/04/21/top-ten-vegetarian-apps-for-apples-iphone offers a list of the best vegetarian apps. One app, Vegan Xpress, finds vegan options at chain restaurants if you're really stuck in the middle of nowhere (or suburbia!).

It can be challenging to travel in foreign countries or very remote areas. Language and cultural preferences can be a barrier. *Vegetarian Passport,* third edition (2010), translates your vegan needs into thirty-three different languages so waiters and food purveyors can help you select the right items. Otherwise, stick with whole fruits and veggies—you may have to cook them in boiling water in certain areas of the world where the water supply may present problems.

Airports are getting better and better at offering healthy and veggie/vegan food, but they still have a long way to go. I wouldn't count on finding a lot of vegan choices in terminal shops and restaurants. And I can't count how many times my preordered in-flight vegan meal wasn't available. So if it's easy to bring your favorite foods with you, stock up, and leave room in your carry-on and suitcase. Bring a salad in a sealed container. I love Dr. Cow cheese (a raw food made from cashews) and crackers. Sea's Gift nori seaweed packs are a great alternative to potato chips.

Traveling light is important, but so is being prepared. I have traveled with a blender in my suitcase—the Magic Bullet is a small blender that is easy to travel with. I also pack protein and green powders with me for shakes, and Baggies of supplements labeled with time of day or meal.

If you can, stay in a hotel room with a kitchenette to prepare your own food or stow farmers' market produce in the fridge. To cook up a feast, access veggie recipes on a smart phone, from your laptop, or from an electronic book reader.

If I am invited to a party or dinner, I always offer to bring my own food so the host doesn't feel obligated to make recipes that may intimidate them or a special meal just for me. Vegan food can sound daunting to people who are new to it. This is a wonderful opportunity for you to introduce people to vegan food, and how good it can taste! If I go to an event and I don't know what's on the menu, I will eat before I leave home.

You can always choose a vegan getaway if you are going on vacation. Check out vegetarian-vacations.com for places and package deals. You can't always plan a trip that way, however. I went to Spain last summer, which isn't the most veggie-friendly place, so I did research and found that their definition of vegetarian isn't quite as strict as ours. They serve chicken at most vegetarian restaurants! But I was able to remain vegan the whole trip by sticking to whole foods (like produce and grains). Gazpacho is a delicious vegan soup!

Remember that being a vegan is adventurous, and so is travel—that sense of exploration, an open mind, and a willingness to be honest about your needs should take you around the world with no problem at all!

Emily Deschanel is star of the Fox series *Bones,* and a health and animal advocate.

Day 17
21-DAY CLEANSE

One of the things I learned on my journey with the little c is that I am my own best friend. And guess what? So are you! When you get to know and respect yourself you are never alone, no matter how hard it gets and how dark it seems. Never forget that, okay? Life is testy. Obstacles are par for the course. Pat yourself on the back! Take pride in how far you've come. You rock!

FOCUS

Now's a good time to ask your best friend (you!):

What needs more attention in your life?

What's one thing you could take off your plate that would allow you more time?

What loving words about yourself would your best friend tell you?

Write those encouraging words on your bathroom mirror in red lipstick.

PRAYER

Obstacles are opportunities in disguise—let me know them when I see them.

AFFIRMATION

I accept and love myself as I am. I believe in me.

GOD POD MAINTENANCE

Get a haircut, invest in some new duds, be Madonna and reinvent yourself. By now you've probably lost a few pounds, your skin looks dewy and youthful, and your attitude shines. Get a style to match the magic.

TIP

Give yourself a belly rub. Your pooper will thank you. Lie on your back with your knees bent, feet on the floor. Apply moderate pressure and slowly rub in a circular clockwise motion. Start on your right side, then work across your belly (under your rib cage) and down your left side. Repeat several times. If you're having trouble with trapped gas, try using a hot-water bottle atop your tum tum.

Day 18
21-DAY CLEANSE

Vision boards help focus our intentions so that we can manifest our desires. I bow to the universal wizardry that is my vision board! If you don't already have one, today is a great time to start one. If you do have a vision board, renovate it. Imbue it with love and reverence, keep it alive and active, and know that it contains major mojo. It's not enough to post stuff and then sit on your sofa and do nothing. Plot and plan your attack! To whet your appetite about all things vision, here's one of my favorite vision board stories. I hope it inspires you.

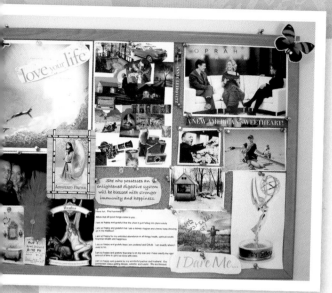

crazy*sexy* CANCER **AND OPRAH**

When I decided to make my film, I wrote the words CRAZY SEXY CANCER on my vision board. Though many network executives told me that I would never get a documentary about cancer (too depressing) with a name like that (too weird) on TV—I did. But I didn't stop there. I tacked an itty-bitty note next to my dream. It read, "Oprah, save a seat for me, I'm coming." Even though I didn't know whether or not I'd be alive, let alone finish a film, I kept my eyes on the prize and poured my heart, soul, and savings into the project. Four years later it aired on TLC and I sat on Lady O's comfy white couch. I don't remember much from that surreal day (other than she liked my perfume and I liked her earrings and she called me a "Crazy Sexy Teacher," which I thought was really cool and she was super-kind and pretty and a great hugger. Oh, and I ate Chinese food when it was all over). "What I know for sure," as Oprah would say, is that I felt a deep sense of pride and

accomplishment that day. When a person is powered by faith, a mission, and a vision board, it's best to get out of their way or you just might get run over.

FOCUS

Creativity! Your tools = scissors, magazines clippings, prayers, quotes, love letters to yourself, glue and poster board or thumb tacks and cork board, and imagination. Let yourself be free to explore anything you desire. Lock your inner editor in the bathroom; she's a damn pain in the ass. When you've created your board, place it where you'll constantly see it. Your vision board doesn't want you to shrink like a violet: it wants you to explode like a thunderous stallion!

PRAYER

Wipe my eyes. Help me see the prosperity and grab the opportunity.

AFFIRMATION

What I wish for is on its way.

GOD POD MAINTENANCE

Belly dance, go to zumba class, take up fencing or tae kwan do. Shake it up. Oh, and are you flossing? A healthy mouth = a healthy body.

TIP

Be French. Yes, you read that right. French women eat small portions. They don't supersize their lives. Leave room for creativity (and Frenchness) by leaving room in your tummy. Eat slowly, know when you're full, and then close up shop.

Day 19
21-DAY CLEANSE

Since we're in the home stretch, we're gonna do something a little different today. Sure, I want you to eat well, affirm, pray, and move. But this assignment—one of my favorite creative writing exercises—takes enormous focus. Write a letter to yourself, but from the perspective of you ten years from now. In it describe how well everything has turned out after ten years. Start your letter with the following words: "You'll never believe what happened!" Put in as many details as you can—where you live, what you look like, how you feel, and what you're doing. Then, share the letter with a friend—that's right—and read it out loud. (Your pal can do it, too.)

Day 20
21-DAY CLEANSE

You are awesome! So how do you feel as the end approaches? Are you excited? Nervous? Inspired? Write about it! Take stock of how far you've come. Notice the lines in your script that you've successfully rewritten. Perhaps a few still need editing. You're near the finish line and it's time for a final push.

FOCUS

Build a Crazy Sexy posse. Create your own sassy support group/wellness stitch-and-bitch. Motivate one another, buddy up, pinkie-swear, and help one another stay on track. It's so much easier to continue this wild ride when you have a pal or two to prod your ass.

PRAYER

May the right people come together to create the most supportive posse imaginable.

AFFIRMATION

I attract supportive and motivating friendships into my life. We love and respect one another. We hold ourselves accountable.

GOD POD MAINTENANCE

Dry brush and use coconut oil on your body after your shower. If you feel like twinkling, check out Simply Divine Botanicals "You Glow Girl" glitter butter. Here are some of the ingredients: glitter (duh!), essential oils, vitamin E, aloe, avocado and shea oil, unconditional love and gratitude.

TIP

Be a Spirulina Ballerina! Spirulina, a blue-green algae, is a good source of B_{12} and iron, as well as a complete protein. This magic green powder builds immunity, helps protect your liver, and is good for digestion. Add some to your smoothie.

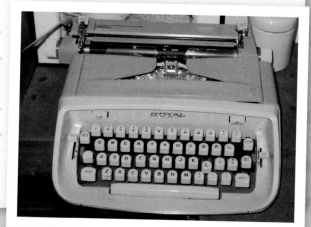

You did it! YEAH! I'm giving you another standing ovation—really—and jumping up and down, too. As you go forward, remember that the Crazy Sexy Diet doesn't have to be all or nothing. Do what you can to stick with an alkaline plant-based diet, feed your soul as well as your body, and pay attention to your inner needs. Write a personal mission statement and let it be your guide. No matter where you are, it will always bring you home. Keep it short and powerful so you remember it always. Place it on your altar. See it, feel it, be it.

MY MISSION STATEMENT

I commit my life to the pursuit of peace. Peace begins with my physical and mental well-being, it extends to my plate, guides all my relationships, personal and business transactions, and decisions. People can't give me happiness; they can only share in my already present happiness stemming from peace.

FOCUS

Live in the present, expect the future.

PRAYER

Knowing I am glorious just as I am, help me face the future with intention, integrity, instinct, and excitement.

AFFIRMATION

I am the embodiment of success today! I am a champion!

GOD POD MAINTENANCE

Ninety-minute deep tissue massage. You deserve it.

TIP

You've changed your diet, moved your ass, unclogged your God pod, prayed Crazy Sexy style, affirmed like a warrior, acknowledged what you love, tapped into the hot spring of gratitude, and possibly even added a pinch of witchcraft "just in case." But what if for some stinking reason you still don't believe in your fabulosity? Well, I got one more trick for ya, act as if. Fake it till you make it. Attitude Olympians have used this training method for generations. Before long you will acknowledge and accept your royalty, without apology. Remember, we successfully manifest our dreams when the feelings behind our intentions are in alignment. Acting as if teaches us to believe in ourselves and never settle for less. When negative, nihilistic thoughts come up, we immediately correct and replace them with positive visualizations and affirmations. "I am sick, weak, and ugly," becomes "I love my body. I am healthy and strong and absolutely stunning." Try on your new confidence until it fits—and go forward.

I love you! Thanks for taking the ride with me, I'm really honored you did . . .

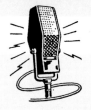

testimonial: Becky B.

After finding Kris's film *Crazy Sexy Cancer* on TLC (okay, I thought the title was weird at first!), I could not help but be drawn to her beautiful soul. Regardless of her state of health, she glowed, and I wanted some of that chutzpah! Suffering from a variety of autoimmune disorders of unknown origins, I was looking for something that Western medicine and the big pharmaceutical companies could not do: Give me my health back now! Or at least give me something that I could do, besides take the Rx and nod obediently. Shortly after the Crazy Sexy Life Web site and community launched, I was hooked. Many changes soon followed: everything from almost entirely eliminating processed foods, sugar, and the usual culprits, to finding friends who have helped me along the way. I've learned and shared my knowledge with anyone and everyone who is in my path. My gastroparesis is better, my thyroid is better, my colitis has healed, and I have grown in more ways than I can count. Now I'm working on my own personal glow from the inside out every day!

Conclusion

Wow, Green Lean God(ess) Machine! We've come a long way in a pretty short time. Bigger news—you just changed your life, even if you've only just started drinking green juices, or tossed the beef and replaced it with beans. How fantastic is that? How brilliant and inspiring are you? Well, I've got a news flash—special alert—the great adventure has only just begun. So many of the people I've met on this journey were just like you before they took the plunge into the CSD pool. Feeling icky—maybe even "suffering" from a disease—and thinking that there's gotta be another way. Hey, I was that person, too! Once you go whole tomato on the diet, and I hope you do, you'll see so many possibilities for your health and happiness. Life gets lighter and you shine brighter. Nice. And when you shake your ass, focus, manifest, pray, and laugh, yowie are you gonna soar. In fact, darlings, I hope you join my online community and tell me your stories and experiences as you continue on the Crazy Sexy path. I can't wait to hear your dish (um, and if you want to send me a new healthy recipe, that's good, too!). Until we meet again, sweet angel . . .

Peace and veggies!

kris carr

Juices and Smoothies

MAKE JUICE, NOT WAR GREEN JUICE

(Serves 2)

It's my motto and my morning beverage. This recipe makes almost 32 ounces.

- 2 large cucumbers (peeled if not organic)
- 4–5 stalks kale
- 4–5 romaine leaves
- 4 stalks celery
- 1–2 big broccoli stems
- 1–2 pears
- 1" piece (or less) gingerroot

Juice all ingredients. Other optional greens: parsley, spinach, and dandelion. Add sweet pea or sunflower sprouts when available.

URBAN ZEN JUICE

Contributed by Marc Alvarez, executive chef, Urban Zen

(Serves 8; 8 cups)

- 6–8 large romaine leaves
- 4–6 leaves lacinato kale
- 2 Granny Smith apples
- 4 Fuji apples
- 1 head fennel
- ½ head celery
- 1 whole cucumber
- 1 yellow pepper
- 1 12-ounce pack baby spinach
- 1" piece gingerroot
- 1 whole lemon

In a large bowl, soak the romaine and kale leaves in cold water. Gently stir the leaves to help remove the sand. Lift the leaves out of the water and place in a new bowl.

Wash the rest of the fruit and vegetables in cold water. Cut all into small pieces that will easily fit into the mouth of the juicer.

Using a Champion Juicer, proceed to juice all of the ingredients, alternating between the leafy vegetables and the fruit. Store in the refrigerator for up to 2 days.

GREEN GURU SMOOTHIE

(Serves 2)

- 1 avocado
- 5–8 romaine leaves
- 1 cucumber
- 2 ounces E3Live
- 1 cup coconut water (or purified water)
- 1 banana or 1–2 pears
- Stevia to taste or 1 teaspoon agave

Place all the ingredients into a blender and blend until smooth.

APPLE SPROUT SMOOTHIE

(Serves 2)

- 1–2 green apples
- 1 small bunch romaine
- 1 cucumber
- ½ tablespoon coconut oil
- 1 cup broccoli or sweet pea sprouts
- Purified water or coconut water
- Stevia to taste or 1 teaspoon agave

Place all the ingredients into a blender and blend until smooth.

WOODSTOCK PEACE SALAD

Use any of the following and dress with
Tahini Dressing

Organic mixed greens (romaine, arugula, or
spinach), diced cucumbers, red peppers, shredded carrots, broccoli florets, diced red onions,
shredded purple cabbage, any sprout (my favorites are sunflower and mung bean sprouts),
avocado, oil-cured olives, and hemp seeds

TAHINI DRESSING

1 cup Tahini

½ cup lemon juice

1 clove garlic

Purified water (use enough to thin out and create desired consistency)

Salt and pepper to taste

Blend all ingredients in a bowl with a whisk until
combined.

TOFU EGGLESS SALAD

Contributed by Chad Sarno, www.rawchef.com

(Serves 6)

2 blocks of firm tofu

1 cup vegan mayonnaise

¼ cup onion, finely diced

½ cup carrot, grated

⅓ cup parsley, finely chopped

¼ cup nutritional yeast

1 tablespoon Dijon mustard

½ teaspoon salt

½ teaspoon pepper

In large bowl, crumble all tofu. Hand mix with
remaining ingredients until thoroughly combined.
Will keep for 5 days.

SHAVED KALE AVOCADO SALAD

Contributed by Chad Sarno, www.rawchef.com

(Serves 2)

1 head kale, shredded

1 cup tomato or red bell pepper, diced

1 cup avocado, chopped

2½ tablespoons olive oil or flax oil

1½ tablespoons lemon juice

1 teaspoon sea salt

½ teaspoon cayenne

In mixing bowl toss all ingredients, squeezing as
you mix to "wilt" the kale and cream the avocado.
Serve immediately.

As a variation, add chopped fresh herbs or your
choice of diced vegetables. You can also substitute
chard or spinach for the kale.

CABBAGE HEMP SALAD

Contributed by Chad Sarno, www.rawchef.com

(Serves 4)

4 cups red or green cabbage, shredded

3 tablespoons hemp or sesame seeds

1½ tablespoons hemp oil

2 tablespoons olive oil

2 tablespoons lemon juice

¼ cup cilantro, chopped

½ tablespoon sea salt

Pinch of cayenne (optional)

In large mixing bowl, toss all ingredients well.
Massage cabbage until dressing is absorbed and
cabbage softens.

VEGAN CAESAR SALAD AND DRESSING

Contributed by Pam Brown, Garden Café, Woodstock, New York, www.gardencafewoodstock.com

- 1 cup Vegenaise
- 1½ teaspoons Dijon mustard
- 1 clove garlic
- 1 tablespoon water
- 1½ teaspoons lemon juice
- 1 tablespoon olive oil
- 1½ teaspoons nutritional yeast
- Salt and pepper to taste

To serve, pour over romaine leaves with chopped red onion. Toast gluten free-bread and cut into small squares for croutons.

MEDITERRANEAN QUINOA SALAD WITH CAPERS

Contributed by Chad Sarno, www.rawchef.com

(Serves 4)

- 3 cups quinoa, cooked
- ¼ cup olive oil
- 3 tablespoons fresh mint or dill, shredded (optional)
- 3 tablespoons capers
- 2 tablespoons lemon juice
- 1 tablespoon lemon zest
- 3 tablespoons pine nuts, lightly toasted
- 3 cloves garlic, minced
- 2 tablespoons leek, finely minced
- Salt and pepper to taste

Hand toss all ingredients; serve warm or chilled.

SIMPLE MEDITERRANEAN SALAD WITH CAPER BERRIES

Contributed by Chad Sarno, www.rawchef.com

(Serves 2)

- 1 cucumber, sliced in thin rounds
- 3 roma tomatoes, sliced thin
- ¼ cup red onion, julienned thin
- ¼ cup caper berries
- 2 tablespoons apple cider vinegar
- 2 tablespoons olive oil
- 3 tablespoons basil, chiffonade
- ½ teaspoon sea salt

Toss all ingredients well. Let stand for an hour to allow flavors to marry before serving.

SWEET DIJON VINAIGRETTE

Contributed by Chad Sarno, www.rawchef.com

(Yields 2 cups)

- ¾ cup prepared Dijon mustard (if using fresh, use a bit less)
- ¾ cup flax oil
- ¼ cup agave nectar
- 2 tablespoons fresh ginger, finely minced
- 4 cloves garlic, finely minced
- ¼ cup apple cider vinegar
- 3 tablespoons shoyu
- ¼ cup water
- 1 tablespoon sea salt

In mixing bowl, whisk all ingredients together until smooth. Add more sweetener to taste.

RAW GREEN GODDESS DRESSING

Contributed by Gena Hamshaw, www.choosingraw.com

(Yields about 1 cup)

¼ cup tahini

¼ cup olive oil

1 tablespoon plus 1 teaspoon nama shoyu

1 teaspoon mellow white miso

2 tablespoons lemon juice

1 teaspoon toasted sesame oil
(not 100 percent raw, but . . .)

2 tablespoons raw and unfiltered apple cider vinegar, such as Bragg's or Eden Organic

1 cup tightly packed parsley

½ cup tightly packed dill

½ cup water

1 clove garlic (optional)

1–2 green onions, chopped (optional)

Blend all the ingredients on high in a food processor, Magic Bullet, or blender (if you're using a food processor, you might want to chop the garlic first).

CARROT MISO DRESSING

Contributed by Gena Hamshaw, www.choosingraw.com

(Makes 3 cups)

3–4 very large carrots (or 7–8 small), chopped

1 cup water

3 tablespoons mellow white miso

1 tablespoon nama shoyu

1 tablespoon lemon juice

3 large, pitted medjool dates

1" piece gingerroot, peeled

1 tablespoon toasted sesame oil

Blend all ingredients save the sesame oil in a Vita-Mix. You'll have to start on low and work the speed up; your machine will sound a little angry, but once it gets blending, it'll simmer down! When you have a creamy, even mix, turn the speed to high and drizzle the sesame oil in. Check the texture: If you'd like it thicker, add some more chopped carrots!

If you don't have a Vita-Mix, simply grate the carrots first, and blend in a conventional blender. Serve on top of a salad or as a dip for some veggie snacking, and enjoy!

AVOCADO CUMIN DRESSING

Contributed by Gena Hamshaw, www.choosingraw.com

(Makes 1 cup)

Inspired by a recipe taught by vegan chef Myra Cornfield, this creamy dressing is always a hit at parties and dinners!

1 teaspoon whole cumin seeds

3 tablespoons fresh lime juice

3 tablespoons extra-virgin olive oil

1 ripe avocado

½ teaspoon salt

½ teaspoon Dijon mustard

1 clove garlic, minced

¼–½ cup water
(depending how thick you like it)

Black pepper

Dry-toast the cumin seeds in a heavy-bottomed skillet until fragrant. Grind into a powder using a spice grinder. Put the ground cumin, lime juice, oil, avocado, salt, mustard, garlic, and water into a blender and blend until very smooth. Sprinkle with pepper and season to taste.

RAW RANCH DRESSING

Contributed by Gena Hamshaw, www.choosingraw .com

(Yields 1½ cups or so)

- ¾ cup cashews, soaked for at least 2 hours
- ½ cup water
- 2 tablespoons lemon juice
- ¼ cup apple cider vinegar (a little more if you like it more tart)
- ¼–½ teaspoon salt
- ½ teaspoon dried thyme
- ½ teaspoon dried oregano
- 1 clove garlic (optional)
- ½ teaspoon onion powder (optional)
- 3 tablespoons fresh dill
- 3 tablespoons fresh parsley
- 3 tablespoons olive oil

Blend all the ingredients in a high-speed blender—or blend all the ingredients except for the oil in a food processor, and drizzle the oil in until the mixture is creamy and emulsified.

When the dressing is blended, chop an additional few tablespoons of herbs and mix them in. Enjoy on top of a big green salad.

GINGERY ASIAN DRESSING

Contributed by Gena Hamshaw, www.choosingraw .com

(Makes 1⅓ cups)

- 1" piece gingerroot (or 1½ teaspoons powdered)
- ½ teaspoon turmeric
- ¾ cup flax oil
- 2 teaspoons sesame oil (toasted)
- ¼ cup lime juice
- 2 tablespoons mellow white miso
- 4 large medjool dates, pitted, or 1–2 packets of stevia
- ¼ cup nama shoyu
- ½ cup water

Blend all ingredients on high till creamy and emulsified.

KING GARLIC HEMP DRESSING

Contributed by Kristen Suzanne, www.kristensraw .com

(Makes 1½ cups)

- 1 cup hemp oil
- ½ cup fresh lemon juice
- 3 large cloves garlic
- 1½ teaspoons Italian seasoning
- ½ teaspoon Himalayan crystal salt

Blend all of the ingredients thoroughly until the mixture reaches a creamy consistency. Drizzle some on your next salad. Stored in an airtight container in your refrigerator, King Garlic Hemp Dressing will stay fresh for up to 5 days.

AZTEC SALAD

Contributed by Candle Café, New York, New York, www.candlecafe.com

(Serves 4)

This rich and satisfying salad is full of the flavors of Mexico. All of the components can be prepared well ahead of time and tossed together just before serving.

FOR THE TEMPEH:

- 8 ounces tempeh, quartered
- 1 cup apple juice
- 1 cup shoyu
- ⅔ cup water
- ¼ cup peeled and shredded ginger
- 2 cloves garlic, minced
- 1 cup agave nectar
- Chipotle Barbecue Sauce (recipe follows)

FOR THE QUINOA:

1½ cups uncooked quinoa

2¾ cups water

1 tablespoon sea salt

2 ears sweet corn, husked

1 red onion, peeled and thinly sliced

1 cup chopped fresh cilantro

1 red bell pepper, seeded, deveined, and cut into thin strips

2 cups dried black beans, cooked and drained, or 2 cups canned beans, drained

Juice of 1 lime

Roasted Tomato Vinaigrette (recipe follows)

FOR THE TOASTED PUMPKIN SEEDS:

1 cup pumpkin seeds

2 teaspoons olive oil

1 teaspoon sea salt

½ teaspoon chili powder

4 cups mesclun

To prepare the tempeh: Preheat the oven to 350 degrees F.

Place the tempeh quarters in a single layer in a baking dish. Mix the apple juice, shoyu, water, ginger, garlic, and agave nectar together and pour over the tempeh. Cover and bake for 45 minutes. Drain the tempeh and let it cool.

Prepare a stovetop or charcoal grill or heat up the broiler. Brush the tempeh with Chipotle Barbecue Sauce and grill until lightly browned.

To prepare the quinoa salad: Rinse the quinoa until the water runs clear, then drain. Bring the water and salt to a boil, add the quinoa, reduce the heat, and simmer. Cover and cook for 20 to 25 minutes. Fluff with a fork and remove the quinoa to a large bowl. Fluff again and set aside to cool.

Cook the corn in boiling salted water for 8 minutes. Drain and cool. Scrape the kernels off the ears with a sharp knife. Set aside.

Toss the onion, cilantro, red pepper, and black beans together. Add the lime juice and toss again.

Mix into the quinoa and gently toss together. Add about ¼ cup Roasted Tomato Vinaigrette and toss again.

To prepare the Toasted Pumpkin Seeds: Preheat the oven to 375 degrees F.

Toss the pumpkin seeds with the olive oil, salt, and chili powder. Spread on a baking sheet and bake until the seeds just begin to pop, 5 to 7 minutes. Set aside to cool.

To assemble the salad: Divide the mesclun into four salad bowls. Place about 1 cup of the dressed quinoa mixture on top of the lettuce. Slice each tempeh square into triangles and place four triangles of tempeh over the quinoa in a spoke pattern. Sprinkle with pumpkin seeds and drizzle with a small amount of dressing.

CHIPOTLE BARBECUE SAUCE

Contributed by Candle Café, New York, New York, www.candlecafe.com

(Makes 5 cups)

This spicy sauce is a great pantry item. We always like to have some on hand to use over grilled tofu or seitan. It's also delicious with grilled vegetables.

3 dried chipotle peppers

3 tablespoons minced garlic

1½ cups tomato paste

1 cup apple cider vinegar

½ cup molasses

1 cup agave nectar

¼ cup mustard

¾ cup dried basil

1 teaspoon sea salt

Freshly ground black pepper

1 cup water

½ cup shoyu

Soak the peppers in hot water for 15 minutes. Drain and chop.

Place the chopped chipotles and the remaining ingredients in a blender and blend until smooth. The sauce will keep, covered, in the refrigerator for up to 2 weeks.

ROASTED TOMATO VINAIGRETTE

Contributed by Candle Café, New York, New York, www.candlecafe.com

(Makes 3 cups)

This is a versatile and delicious dressing. Its robust flavor holds up to a variety of vegetables and grains, as well as salads.

- 4 Roma tomatoes, halved
- 1¼ cups plus 1 tablespoon extra-virgin olive oil
- ½ teaspoon sea salt
- Freshly ground black pepper
- ½ cup red wine vinegar
- 1 teaspoon crushed red pepper flakes
- 2 cloves garlic, minced
- 2 tablespoons chopped fresh cilantro

Preheat the oven to 400 degrees F.

Toss the tomatoes with 1 tablespoon of the olive oil, along with the salt and pepper. Place the tomatoes on a baking sheet, cut-side down, and roast for 20 to 25 minutes, until the skin blisters. Set aside to cool.

Transfer the tomatoes, remaining 1¼ cups olive oil, vinegar, red pepper flakes, garlic, cilantro, and salt and pepper to a blender and blend until smooth. Taste and adjust the seasonings. The vinaigrette will keep, covered, in the refrigerator for up to a week.

Variation: For a Spicy Southwestern-Style Roasted Tomato Vinaigrette, add 4 rehydrated chipotles to the tomatoes before blending.

TUNISIAN KALE SALAD WITH OLIVES AND LEMONY RAW TAHINI DRESSING

Contributed by Latham Thomas, Tender Shoots Wellness, www.tendershootswellness.com

(Serves 8)

- 2½ bunches dino kale (lacinato), cut in thin strips across ribs
- 1 teaspoon sea salt
- ¼ cup extra-virgin olive oil
- ¼ cup (2 ounces) nama shoyu
- 1 tablespoon raw agave nectar
- 1 teaspoon spicy curry
- ½ cup lemon juice
- 1 teaspoon cayenne pepper
- 1 cup raw tahini
- 1 ounce grated gingerroot
- 1 cup pine nuts
- 1½ cups pitted green olives
- 1½ cups diced red bell pepper
- 1 cup hemp seeds

Take 3 stalks of kale and stack together. Slice the kale in ¼-inch ribbons across the ribs to get thin slices. Blend all the other ingredients (minus the olives, bell pepper, and hemp seeds) to get a thick dressing. Add the olives, bell pepper, and hemp seeds to the bowl with kale. Then pour over the tahini dressing and mix thoroughly. Allow the kale to wilt when mixed with the dressing—the salt and acid from lemon in the dressing softens the kale and makes the fiber more tender and easier to digest. Massaging the kale is a part of it as well, so use a nice wooden spoon or your own hands to mix.

This salad can be served right away or made a day ahead. It won't keep very long in the fridge if dressed—maybe 2 days tops before it gets soggy. Prepping for a few days ahead? Keep the kale and dressing separate and dress prior to serving.

TOMATO WILD RICE SOUP

Contributed by Chad Sarno, www.rawchef.com

(Serves 4)

½ cup sun-dried tomatoes, soaked in water

1 tablespoon garlic, minced

3 cups water (preferably water used to soak sun-dried tomatoes)

3 cups tomato, chopped

½ cup parsley, chopped

⅓ cup basil, chopped

1 zucchini, chopped

½ apple

2 tablespoons fresh oregano, minced

½ tablespoon sea salt

¼ teaspoon cayenne or minced hot chile pepper

Dash white pepper

2 cups wild rice, sprouted

1½ cups diced portobello mushrooms, marinated in 2 tablespoons nama shoyu

In Vita-Mix blend sun-dried tomatoes, garlic, and 1 cup water until smooth. Add all remaining ingredients except rice and mushrooms. Blend on low to a slightly chunky consistency. Add rice and mushrooms and blend on low for 10–20 seconds. Serve warm.

RAW GODDESS SOUP

(Serves 1–2)

1 large avocado

1 red pepper

2 cups salad greens

Handful of kale

1–2 scallions

1 teaspoon dulse

Sea salt or Bragg's apple cider to taste

1 clove garlic, crushed

Pinch of cayenne

Fresh herbs like dill, thyme, and basil to taste

Purified water

Blend all ingredients. Use purified water to thin it out. You don't have to follow this recipe exactly—what veggies do you love? You can also use olive oil or flax oil in place of the avocado.

MISO BROTH WITH ZUCCHINI SOMEN AND SHIITAKE

Contributed by Chad Sarno, www.rawchef.com

(Serves 4)

¼ cup dark barley miso

4 cups warm water

1½ tablespoons fresh ginger, chopped

2 cloves garlic

2 tablespoons sesame oil

½ tablespoon shoyu

¼ teaspoon cayenne

1 zucchini, peeled and spiralized using spiral slicer

8–9 shiitake mushrooms, stems removed, sliced paper thin, and marinated in 1 tablespoon shoyu and 1 tablespoon olive oil

2 tablespoons green onion, finely diced

In high speed blender, liquefy the miso, warm water, ginger, garlic, sesame oil, shoyu, and cayenne. Pour soup slowly through a fine mesh strainer, being sure not to create foam. To serve, pour into bowls and top with equal parts of the remaining ingredients. Serve warm.

GINGER-LEMONGRASS MISO SOUP

Contributed by Candle Café, New York, New York, www.candlecafe.com

(Serves 6–8)

Lemongrass, an important ingredient in Thai cooking, adds a wonderful, refreshing flavor to soup, especially when combined with miso and ginger. Serve this delicious and revitalizing soup with a salad and grains.

- 8 cups water
- 1 stalk lemongrass, trimmed, peeled, and thinly sliced
- 1 teaspoon sesame oil
- 1 cup yellow onion, peeled, halved and thinly sliced
- 2 tablespoons minced gingerroot
- ¾ cup white miso
- 1 cup enoki mushrooms, for garnish
- 1 cup thinly sliced scallions (green part only), for garnish

Bring the water and lemongrass to a boil and simmer for 15 minutes; discard the lemongrass and strain, reserving the water.

Heat the oil in a sauté pan and cook the onion and ginger until the onion is translucent, about 10 minutes. Transfer to a soup pot and add the reserved water; bring to a boil, reduce the heat, and simmer, uncovered, for 5 minutes. Turn off heat and stir in the miso.

Ladle the soup into bowls, garnish with enoki mushrooms and scallions, and serve immediately.

LIVE CUCUMBER AND AVOCADO SOUP

Contributed by Angel Ramos, executive chef, Candle 79, New York, New York, www.candle79.com

(Serves 6–8)

- 8 cucumbers, roughly chopped
- 4 avocados, peels and pits removed
- 1 jalapeño, seeds removed
- ½ bunch cilantro
- 1 sprig mint, stems removed
- 1 lime, juiced
- 2 tablespoons salt
- 1 small radish, julienned and chopped
- ½ red bell pepper, julienned and chopped
- Sweet corn kernels cut from 1 ear

In a high-speed blender, combine the cucumbers, avocados, jalapeño, cilantro, mint leaves, lime juice, and salt. Blend on high until all ingredients have been well pureed (about 1 to 2 minutes).

Place a chinois (china cap) over a 1- or 2-quart container. Pass the puree through the chinois, working it through with a spatula if necessary. Taste and reseason if desired.

Ladle a serving of the cucumber and avocado soup into a bowl. Place the julienne of radish and red pepper, and some sweet corn kernels on top to garnish. Enjoy!

KRISTEN SUZANNE'S HARVEST SOUP

Contributed by Kristen Suzanne, www.kristensraw.com

(Makes 6 cups)

1 cup water

1 large zucchini, chopped

2 medium tomatoes, quartered

3 stalks celery, chopped

2 cups carrot, chopped

2 dates, pitted

1 clove garlic

2 teaspoons Himalayan crystal salt

1 tablespoon onion powder

½ teaspoon black pepper

½ cup flax oil or olive oil

Fun Variations:

Add ½ teaspoon coriander

Add ½ teaspoon pumpkin pie spice

Blend all of the ingredients, except for the oil, on high speed in your blender until really creamy (approximately 1 minute—I prefer this soup a tad warm and very creamy). Then, while the blender is running on low speed, add the oil. Continue blending, at a higher speed, for another minute or less. Enjoy!

Sauces

PRANA MARINARA SAUCE

(Serves 2)

1 cup cherry tomatoes

1 yellow bell pepper

¼ cup sun-dried tomatoes

1 cup basil

1 tablespoon olive oil

Sea salt to taste

Dried thyme to taste

Dried oregano to taste

Blend all ingredients in a high-speed blender till thick and smooth.

ELECTRIC LOTUS PESTO

(Serves 2)

2 cups tightly packed basil leaves

2 cloves garlic

½ teaspoon sea salt

½ cup pine nuts

½ cup olive oil

Place all ingredients in a food processor (or blender) and blend until smooth.

Serve pasta sauces over gluten-free noodles made from zucchini or squash. To make raw noodles you'll need a spiral slicer (amazon.com).

Main Courses

I AM LOVED NORI ROLLS
(Serves 3–4)

- 4 nori seaweed sheets
- 2–3 cups of cooked short grain brown rice
- Tahini
- ½ cucumber, sliced thinly into sticks
- 1 small carrot, sliced thinly into sticks
- ½ avocado, julienned
- 2 scallions, sliced thinly into sticks
- ½ cup sunflower sprouts
- Bragg's Liquid Aminos, or gluten-free nama shoyu or tamari
- ¼ cup grated ginger juice

Place a sheet of nori shiny-side down on a bamboo mat. Work with wet hands and keep a small bowl of water nearby to dip your fingers in. Spread a thin layer of the rice evenly over the nori, leaving about ½ inch on the top edge. Spread a very thin layer of tahini over the rice. Place 2 strips of cucumber at the end closest to you. Leave about 1 inch from the bottom. Next to it add ¼ of the carrot, avocado, and scallions. Sprinkle a few sprouts on top. Roll the nori tightly from the bottom, using the mat to help make it tight. Seal it with a few drops of water on the ½ inch of nori at the top.

Carefully slice the roll into inch-thick rounds. Use a serrated knife dipped in a tiny bit of water. Repeat with the remaining ingredients. Dip in Bragg's Liquid Aminos or gluten-free nama shoyu. Add the juice of grated ginger to the sauce to give it a kick!

You can also make raw nori rolls by using jicama, cauliflower, or turnip in place of rice. Use a food processor to chop the veggies so that they look grainy.

BUDDHA BOWL
(Serves 2–3)

Buddha Bowls are fast food for the conscious eater. Use any combo of slightly steamed, sautéed, or finely chopped raw veggies on top of a gluten-free grain (millet, quinoa, brown rice, what have you). Add an avocado to up the yum factor.

Here's an example that serves 2 hungry people.

- 1–2 cups of brown rice (you'll have extra)
- ½ head broccoli
- 1 cup chickpeas
- ½ purple onion, diced
- 1 grated carrot
- 1 clove garlic
- ¼ cup ground flaxseeds
- ¼ cup hemp seeds
- 1 avocado
- ½ cup diced oil-cured olives
- Sea salt or Bragg's to taste (olives are salty so go easy)
- 1 tablespoon olive oil or flax oil (optional)
- Dash of cayenne

Cook the brown rice first. Use a 2:1 ratio of water to rice in the cooking process. If you're using raw veggies, finely chop them and toss them with the rice while it's still hot. This cooks them a bit, but you don't lose nutrients. Season and dress to taste.

SEXY SEED CAKES
(Servings vary depending on size of cakes)

- ¼ cup raw pumpkin seeds
- ¼ cup raw sunflower seeds
- ¼ cup raw flaxseeds
- ¼ cup raw sesame seeds or hemp seeds
- 1 cup ground millet or gluten-free flour
- 1½ teaspoons baking soda

½ teaspoon sea salt

1 packet (or more) stevia

Pinch of cinnamon

Unsweetened hemp milk to thin batter

Use a coffee grinder for all the seeds except the hemp—they don't need to be ground. Use the grinder for the millet as well, or just use gluten-free flour. Mix all the ingredients with passion. Pour heaping tablespoons of batter onto a hot pan or griddle coated with coconut oil—the best oil for high heat. Cook until the batter starts to bubble and flip when the bottom of the cake is slightly brown. Finish with a drizzle of agave and serve.

THAI "PEANUT" SAUCE VEGETABLES

Contributed by Chad Sarno, www.rawchef.com

(Serves 4)

½ cup almond butter

1 tablespoon fresh ginger, chopped

1½ tablespoons lemon juice

2 tablespoons sweetener (dates, raisins, or prunes)

2 cloves garlic

1½ tablespoons sea salt or 1½ tablespoons shoyu

1 teaspoon serrano pepper, diced (optional)

⅓ cup water, plus more to thin sauce

2 zucchini, sliced in half moons

2 carrots, julienned

1 cup broccoli florets

1 cup snow peas

½ cup cilantro, chopped

In high speed blender, blend the almond butter, ginger, lemon juice, sweetener, garlic, salt, serrano pepper, and water until smooth. Add water as needed to achieve desired thickness. Toss the sauce with vegetables and cilantro in large mixing bowl.

When vegetables are tossed well, dehydrate on Teflex sheets at 105 degrees for 2–3 hours to soften.

MEXICAN PILAF

Contributed by Chad Sarno, www.rawchef.com

(Serves 4)

3 cups wild rice, sprouted or cooked

3 tablespoons green onion, diced

1½ cups tomato, diced

½ cup cilantro, chopped

2 tablespoons fresh oregano, minced

½ cup sun-dried tomatoes, soaked 1–3 hours

1½ tablespoons white miso

1 tablespoon garlic, minced

1 tablespoon chili powder

½ teaspoon cumin

2 tablespoons lemon juice

3 tablespoons olive oil

1 teaspoon sea salt

Place sprouted or cooked rice in mixing bowl and hand toss with the green onion, 1 cup diced tomato, cilantro, and oregano. Set aside. In high speed blender, blend the sun-dried tomatoes, remaining ½ cup diced tomato, miso, garlic, chili powder, cumin, lemon juice, olive oil, and salt until smooth. Toss tomato paste with rice and mix well.

SOUTHWEST BLACK BEAN AND ROASTED SWEET POTATO BURGER

Contributed by Pam Brown, Garden Café, Woodstock, New York, www.gardencafewoodstock.com

(Makes 10 patties)

2 cups cooked black beans, mashed

Sweet potatoes to equal 2 cups when peeled and cut into small cubes

2 teaspoons olive oil

Salt

3 ounces yellow onion, diced

2 teaspoons garlic

3 tablespoons tamari

2 teaspoons ground cumin

Pepper

7 ounces cooked rice

1½ teaspoons vegetarian Worcestershire sauce

1 ounce cornmeal, plus 1 ounce for dredging

Preheat the oven to 350 degrees F.

Place the mashed black beans in a bowl. Peel and cut the sweet potatoes, dropping them in cold water as you cut them. Drain well and toss with olive oil and salt. Spread them out in an even layer on a lightly oiled baking sheet. Roast in the oven for 25 to 30 minutes, or until tender. Toss occasionally.

Heat a bit of olive oil in a large sauté pan over medium high heat. Add the onion and garlic and cook until lightly browned. Add the onions to the bowl of beans. Stir in the tamari, cumin, and salt and pepper to taste. Add the cooked rice, sweet potatoes, Worcestershire sauce, and 1 ounce of cornmeal. Mix well and adjust the seasonings. Form into 4½-ounce patties and dredge lightly in the remaining 1 ounce of cornmeal. Heat a cast-iron skillet over medium heat and add more olive oil. Add the burgers and brown lightly on each side. Place on a baking sheet and bake for 10 minutes.

Serve with salsa and guacamole on your favorite bun or bread.

OLIVE QUESADILLAS

Contributed by Pam Brown, Garden Café, Woodstock, New York, www.gardencafewoodstock.com

(Serves 1–2)

1 large flour tortilla

4 ounces Follow Your Heart vegan cheese or Daiya cheese

2 ounces caramelized onions

2 ounces roasted red peppers

8 kalamata olives, halved

Spread cheese on one half of the tortilla. Add the onions, peppers, and olives evenly. Fold the tortilla over and grill until it's golden and crispy.

CHOOSING RAW "PEANUT" NOODLES

Contributed by Gena Hamshaw, www.choosingraw.com

(Serves 1–2)

FOR THE ASIAN DRESSING:

(Makes 1½ cups)

1" piece gingerroot

1 cup olive oil (or flax oil)

2 teaspoons toasted sesame oil

Juice of 1 lime

¼ cup mellow white miso

6 dates, pitted, or ¼ cup maple syrup

2 tablespoons nama shoyu

⅓ cup water

Blend all ingredients on high till creamy and emulsified.

FOR THE NOODLES:

1 large or 2 small zucchinis, spiralized or sliced with a vegetable peeler

½ red pepper, sliced into matchsticks

½ carrot, sliced into matchsticks

¼ large or ½ small cucumber, grated or peeled into long strips

Scallions or green onion to garnish

To make the dish, simply prepare and mix all veg-gies, save the scallions or green onion. Toss them with ¼ cup dressing, adding more if necessary, and sprinkle with scallions.

Sugar snaps, shiitake mushrooms, snow pea shoots, or mung bean sprouts would also be a great addition to the noodles.

TERIYAKI TOFU

Contributed by Chad Sarno, www.rawchef.com

(Serves 4)

2 blocks of tofu, each in 6 slices

3 tablespoons shoyu or tamari

1 tablespoon sesame oil

½ cup pineapple juice

3 tablespoons rice vinegar

2 tablespoons agave syrup

2 cloves garlic, minced

1 tablespoon ginger, finely minced

½ teaspoon hot chile pepper, minced

In mixing bowl, whisk all ingredients except tofu well. Pour marinade into container, submerge sliced tofu, and allow to sit 1–3 hours.

Place tofu on baking sheet and pour ¼ of the mar-inade over it. Slow bake the tofu at 300 degrees for 1–1½ hours, flipping halfway through. It's done when marinade is evaporated and tofu is firm. Serve with chilled buckwheat noodles.

ROASTED TOMATOES STUFFED WITH PINE NUT SPINACH PÂTÉ AND YOUNG DILL

Contributed by Chad Sarno, www.rawchef.com

(Yields 4 cups or stuffing for 8–10 tomatoes)

1½ cups pine nuts

2 cloves garlic

2 tablespoons lemon juice

⅓ cup water

1 teaspoon nutmeg

½ teaspoon sea salt

2 tablespoons olive oil

1½ cups red bell pepper, diced

1 cup sun-dried black olives, pitted and minced

2 tablespoons fresh basil, minced

3 tablespoons fresh dill, minced

1½ tablespoons fresh oregano, minced

1½ cups baby spinach, shredded

8–10 tomatoes, roasted and with pulp scooped out to make cups

In a food processor, process the pine nuts, garlic, lemon juice, water, nutmeg, salt, and olive oil until smooth. Remove to a mixing bowl and hand mix with remaining ingredients, except tomatoes. Stuff tomatoes with mixture.

ASIAN MEDLEY (AKA STIR RAW)

Contributed by Chad Sarno, www.rawchef.com

(Serves 4–6)

1 cup broccoli florets

1 cup red bell pepper, julienned

1 cup red cabbage, shredded

1 cup carrots, julienned thin

1 cup portobello mushrooms, cubed and mari-nated in 3 tablespoons olive oil and 2 table-spoons nama shoyu

1 cup Asian bean sprouts

½ cup cilantro, chopped

½ cup fresh basil, torn

½ cup olive oil

⅔ cup orange juice

3 tablespoons white miso

2 tablespoons nama shoyu

3 tablespoons fresh ginger, chopped

1 tablespoon garlic, minced

½ tablespoon sea salt

1 teaspoon cayenne

In large bowl, toss the broccoli, bell pepper, cabbage, carrot, marinated portobello mushrooms, asian bean sprouts, cilantro, and basil. Set aside.

In high speed blender, blend olive oil, orange juice, miso, shoyu, ginger, garlic, salt, and cayenne. Toss the sauce with the mixture of vegetables. Allow to marinate for about an hour. Spread on Teflex sheet on dehydrator tray and dehydrate at 105 degrees for 1 hour. Serve warm.

PALAK PANEER (SPINACH W/ CREAM SAUCE)

Contributed by Chad Sarno, www.rawchef.com

(Serves 4)

½ cup pine nuts

1½ tablespoons lemon juice

2 tablespoons olive oil

½ tablespoon garlic

1 tablespoon fresh ginger, finely minced

1 tablespoon garam masala

½ teaspoon cinnamon

¼ teaspoon black pepper

1 teaspoon salt

4 cups baby spinach

¼ cup red bell pepper, diced

3 tablespoons chives, minced

In high speed blender, blend the pine nuts, lemon juice, olive oil, garlic, ginger, garam masala, cinnamon, pepper, and salt until smooth. Mix in the baby spinach, diced bell pepper, and chives by hand. You can choose to warm by placing on a dehydrator sheet at 105 degrees for 1 hour.

MARINATED SEA VEGETABLES

Contributed by Chad Sarno, www.rawchef.com

(Serves 4)

2 cups arame, rehydrated

2 cups hijiki, rehydrated

3 tablespoons green onions, finely diced

1 tablespoon nama shoyu

2 tablespoons olive oil

1 tablespoon fresh lime juice

½ teaspoon toasted sesame oil

3 tablespoons white sesame seeds

In mixing bowl toss all ingredients well. Serve immediately or store in refrigerator.

Desserts

AVOCADO CHOCOLATE PUDDING (AKA CHOCOMOLE!)

Contributed by Gena Hamshaw, www.choosingraw.com

- 1 ripe avocado, pitted
- 6–10 dates (depending on size of dates), soaked if necessary
- ½ teaspoon vanilla
- 4 heaping tablespoons cocoa or 2 tablespoons carob powder
- ½ cup water

Place the first four ingredients in a food processor (you can use a blender or Vita-Mix, but food processors work much better for this recipe) and begin blending.

Drizzle in the water, stopping to scrape the sides of the bowl if need be, until the mixture resembles a thick chocolate pudding. Let it continue mixing until smooth and creamy. If you are on a low-glycemic or anti-candida diet, use stevia or agave to taste in place of the dates.

VANILLA CHIA TAPIOCA PUDDING

Contributed by Latham Thomas, Tender Shoots Wellness, www.tendershootswellness.com

- 7 cups milk (brazil nut, hemp seed, or cashew)
- 2 tablespoons vanilla extract
- 1 vanilla bean
- 2 tablespoons cinnamon
- ⅓ cup agave nectar
- Pinch of sea salt
- 1 cup chia seeds

Blend all the ingredients (minus the chia seeds) in a high-speed blender and pulse. Place the chia seeds in a large bowl, pour the mixture over them, and begin to whisk. Keep whisking periodically to be sure the tapioca does not clump. It takes about an hour and a half for the tapioca to set. You can adjust the sweetness. This is great for a healthy omega-rich quick dessert or a kids' snack.

BANANA SOFT SERVE

Contributed by Gena Hamshaw, choosingraw.com

Take 2 or 3 frozen bananas (you can freeze them in resealable bags or in Tupperware) and throw them in your food processor. Then turn the processor on and let it run for about 5 minutes, stopping every now and then to scrape down the sides. The bananas should get increasingly light, fluffy, and smooth. By the time you're done, they'll resemble a creamy bowl of soft serve. Scoop them into a bowl and prepare to marvel!

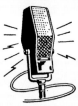

testimonial: Jody L.

After trying the Crazy Sexy Diet, I believe I can fly! (Cape not included.) I literally feel like I have a new lease on life. Prior to starting the cleanse, I was desperately searching for a remedy to my "funk" (depression). Upon doing a search on the Internet and stumbling upon crazysexylife.com, the timing couldn't have been more appropriate. Joining the community and taking the initiative to participate in the cleanse—that was my first baby step of taking control of my life. It brings me to tears (of joy) to feel the way I do now. After cutting dairy out of my diet, I felt so much better spirit-wise, and no more gross mucus in the morning upon waking up. The refined foods, wheat, and gluten are hasta la vista, baby! I don't have bloating anymore. I don't have any cravings for meat, chicken, or fish. Juicing and creating new raw meals have become a fun introduction to food. To sum things up, I am back and proud to call myself VEGAN.

crazy sexy RESOURCES

BOOKS

DIET AND LIFESTYLE

Anticancer: A New Way of Life by David Servan-Schreiber, MD

Becoming Raw: The Essential Guide to Raw Vegan Diets by Brenda Davis, RD, and Vesanto Melina, MS, RD

Becoming Vegan by Brenda Davis, RD, and Vesanto Melina, MS, RD

The Body Ecology Diet: Recovering Your Health and Rebuilding Your Immunity by Donna Gates with Linda Schatz

The China Study by T. Colin Campbell, PhD, and Thomas M. Campbell II

Clean by Alejandro Junger, MD

Colon Health by Dr. Norman W. Walker

Conscious Eating by Gabriel Cousens, MD

Crazy Sexy Cancer Survivor: More Rebellion and Fire for Your Healing Journey by Kris Carr

Crazy Sexy Cancer Tips by Kris Carr

The Detox Strategy by Brenda Watson and Leonard Smith

Dr. Neal Barnard's Program for Reversing Diabetes by Neal D. Barnard, MD

Eat Right America by Dr. Joel Fuhrman

Food for Life: How the New Four Food Groups Can Save Your Life by Neal D. Barnard, MD

The Food Revolution by John Robbins

Gluten-Free Diet by Shelley Case

Healing the New Childhood Epidemics: Autism, ADHD, Asthma, and Allergies: The Groundbreaking Program for the 4-A Disorders by Kenneth Bock, MD

The Hundred-Year Lie: How Food and Medicine Are Destroying Your Health by Randall Fitzgerald

In Defense of Food: An Eater's Manifesto by Michael Pollan

The Life Force Diet by Michelle Schoffro Cook

Life Over Cancer: The Block Center Program for Integrative Cancer Treatment by Keith Block, MD

Living Foods for Optimum Health by Theresa Foy Digeronimo and Brian R. Clement

The Mucusless Diet Healing System by Arnold Ehret

Quantum Wellness by Kathy Freston

Revive: Stop Feeling Spent and Start Living Again by Frank Lipman, MD

Skinny Bitch by Rory Freedman and Kim Barnouin

The Spectrum: A Scientifically Proven Program to Feel Better, Live Longer, Lose Weight, and Gain Health by Dean Ornish, MD

UltraMind Solution: Fix Your Broken Brain by Healing Your Body First by Mark Hyman, MD

World Peace Diet by Will Tuttle, PhD

Yoga and Vegetarianism by Sharon Gannon and Ingrid Newkirk

ENZYMES

The Enzyme Factor by Hiromi Shinya, MD

Enzyme Nutrition by Dr. Edward Howell

Everything You Need to Know About Enzymes by Tom Bohager

FOOD COMBINING

The Complete Book of Food Combining by Kathryn Marsden

Fit for Life by Harvey Diamond and Marilyn Diamond

Food Combining and Digestion by Steve Meyerowitz

GLYCEMIC INDEX

The GI Handbook by Barbara Ravage

The New Glucose Revolution: Low GI Eating Made Easy by Jennie Brand-Miller, MD, Kaye Foster-Powell, and Philippa Sandall

JUICING AND FASTING

The Complete Book of Juicing by Michael T. Murray, ND

Fresh Vegetable and Fruit Juices by Dr. Norman Walker

Juicing for Life by Cherie Calbom

The Wheatgrass Book by Ann Wigmore

pH

The Acid–Alkaline Diet for Optimum Health by Christopher Vasey and Jon Graham

The pH Miracle by Dr. Robert O. Young and Shelley Redford Young

The Ultimate pH Solution by Michelle Schoffro Cook

RECIPES, COOKED

The Candle Cafe Cookbook: More than 150 Recipes from New York's Renowned Vegan Restaurant by Joy Pierson, Bart Potenza, and Barbara Scott-Goodman

The Conscious Cook by Tal Ronnen

The Gluten-Free Vegan by Susan O'Brien

The Real Food Daily Cookbook: Really Fresh, Really Good, Really Vegetarian by Ann Gentry

The Ultimate Uncheese Cookbook by Jo Stepaniak

Veganomicon by Isa Chandra Moskowitz and Terry Hope Romero

The Vegan Table: 200 Unforgettable Recipes for Entertaining Every Guest at Every Occasion by Colleen Patrick-Goudreau

RECIPES, RAW

Ani's Raw Food Kitchen: Easy, Delectable Living Foods Recipes by Ani Phyo

Everyday Raw by Matthew Kenney

I Am Grateful: Recipes and Lifestyle of Café Gratitude by Terces Engelhart

Living in the Raw by Rose Lee Calabro

Living on Live Food by Alissa Cohen

Raw Food Real World: 100 Recipes to Get the Glow by Matthew Kenney and Sarma Melngailis

The Raw Gourmet by Nomi Shannon

WEB SITES

ANIMAL WELFARE

ASPCA: www.aspca.org

Farm Sanctuary: www.farm sanctuary.org

Humane Society: www.humane society.org

PETA: www.peta.org

COLON THERAPISTS

The Colon Therapists Network: www.colonhealth.net/ therapist-search

International Association of Colon Therapists: www.i-act.org

COMMUNITY-SUPPORTED AGRICULTURE (csa)

Biodynamic Farming and Gardening Association: www.bio dynamics.com/csa1.html

Local Harvest: www.localharvest .org

National Sustainable Agriculture Information Service: http://attra .ncat.org/attra-pub/local_food

CONSUMER SAFETY

Air Purifiers: www.air-purifiers-america.com

Campaign for Safe Cosmetics: www.safecosmetics.org

Environmental Working Group: www.ewg.org

Food and Water Watch: www .foodandwaterwatch.org

The Guide to Less Toxic Products: lesstoxicguide.ca

Ionized water: www.jupiter ionizers.com, kanganwater usa.com

Skin Deep: www.cosmetics database.com

Water filtration systems: www .wellnessfilter.com

CO-OPS

Co-op Directory Service: www .coopdirectory.org/directory.htm

Cooperative Grocer: www .cooperativegrocer.coop/coops

Local Harvest: www.localharvest .org

DETOX CENTERS

Ann Wigmore Natural Health Institute: www.annwigmore.org

Hippocrates Health Institute: www.hippocratesinst.org

Living Foods Institute: www.living foodsinstitute.com

Optimum Health Institute: www .optimumhealth.org

Tree of Life Rejuvenation Center: www.treeoflife.nu

We Care Spa: www.wecarespa .com

FARMERS' MARKETS

Farmers Market dot com: http:// farmersmarket.com

Farmers Market Online: www .farmersmarketonline.com/Open air.htm

Local Harvest: www.localharvest .org

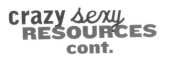

GLUTEN-FREE

Celiac Chicks: www.celiacchicks
.com

Celiac Disease Foundation: www
.celiac.org

Celiac.com: www.celiac
.com/catalog/product_info
.php?products_id=467

The Gluten Free Casein Free Diet:
www.gfcfdiet.com

NATURAL FOOD HOME DELIVERY

Diamond Organics: www
.diamondorganics.com

Frontier Natural Brands: www
.frontiercoop.com

Gold Mine Natural Foods: www
.goldminenaturalfoods.com

Jaffe Bros. Natural Foods: www
.organicfruitsandnuts.com

RAW FOOD HUBS

Choosing Raw: www.choosingraw
.com

Kristen's Raw: www.kristensraw
.com

We Like It Raw: www.welikeitraw
.com

VEGAN, VEGETARIAN, AND RAW RESTAURANTS

Happy Cow: www.happycow.net/

Veg Dining: www.vegdining.com/
Home.cfm

Vegetarian-Restaurants.net: www
.vegetarian-restaurants.net/usa/
index.html

www.allrawdirectory.com
/rawfoods.asp?topic
=rawfoodrestaurants

VEGAN/VEGETARIAN INFORMATION

Choose Veg: http://chooseveg.com

PCRM: www.pcrm.org

T. Colin Campbell: www.tcolin
campbell.org

The Vegetarian Resource Group:
www.vrg.org

Vegan MD: http://veganmd.com

WATER

Clean Water Action: www.clean
wateraction.org/Guide to Tap
Water Filtration

Food and Water Watch: www
.foodandwaterwatch.org/
take-action/consumer-tools/
choosing-a-water-filter

WellOwner.org: www.wellowner
.org

WHEATGRASS DELIVERY

Perfect Foods:
www.800wheatgrass.com

Sproutman: www.sproutman.com

Wheatgrass Central: www.wheat
grasscentral.com

acknowledgments

Thanks:

To all my teachers, without you I would still be eating, drinking, and thinking crap!

To my brilliant posse for their cutting-edge wisdom, passion, and activism.

To Mehmet Oz for his heartfelt guidance and generous support of my work.

To Dean Ornish for being Dean Ornish! Thank you for reminding me to trust my gut.

To my unicorn soul mate Rory Freedman for the kick-ass preface. Nana loves you.

To Neal Barnard, MD, and Jill Eckart. Thank you for believing in me and for helping me move mountains.

To Chad Sarno for creating many of the recipes for the cleanse. Thank you for your culinary genius and for being a really cool dude and visionary.

To all the other contributing chefs for teaching us that delicious can also be healthy.

To my dear friends at Candle 79—Joy Pierson, Bart Potenza, and Benay Vynerib. Thank you for your endless support and for filling my tummy with healing food.

To Sheila Buff for her wonderful research and nutritional expertise.

To Karen Kelly for helping me pull it all together with solid edits and a dash of fairy dust.

To Mary Norris for believing in me for a third charm-filled time around.

To Gena Hamshaw for validating my work and giving me the confidence to put it out there with pride.

To Jennifer Reilly, RD, for fact checking all of my research and giving it her gold star stamp of approval.

To my agent Maura Teitelbaum for being part goddess, part lioness. Someday I'll buy you a house in Boca (or rent one for a weekend depending on how this book thing goes).

To Karla Baker for her feisty and fabulous designs that make my books delightfully accessible. I hope we work together for a long time.

To the talented Victor Juhasz for his wonderful illustration of an unhappy world.

To all the photographers who shared their gorgeous work and talent, especially Alysia Cotter, David Sax, Clif Bumford, Bob Esposito, and Rick Lew.

To our best friends Mary and Ryan Giuliani for letting me shoot in their gorgeous Woodstock home.

To the Humane Society and Farm Sanctuary for supplying the sobering images of what really happens on soul-crushing factory farms.

To my dear friend Kathy Stevens at the Catskill Animal Sanctuary for supplying many of the inspiring images of her soul-ful farm animals. Thank you for rescuing these individuals.

To wild and wonderful Jenny Brown at the Woodstock Farm Animal Sanctuary. Thank you for the beautiful cow and pig images. (Please visit and support both of these farms!)

To Steve Heller for allowing me to shoot his fabulous rocket ship art.

To Corinne Bowen, a brilliant writer, a creative tour de force, my right and left hand and cherished friend. Doing what I do is so much better with you. I love you to the marrow.

To Thomas (T-paw) the cat for being Corinne's industrious intern and confidant.

To Jan Fine, Lola's godmother and our great pal. Thank you for making my furry daughter's life fun and adventurous while I sat in front of my computer for two years.

To Lola for being the best rescue dog and a great example of why people should adopt. I love you so much it hurts my teeth.

To my parents, sister, and husband for standing by my side, supporting and loving me.

To Joni Mitchell, the Beatles, Euphoria, the Band, Bob Dylan, Corinne Bailey Rae, Yo-Yo Ma, Krishna Das, Eddie Vedder, Donna De Lory, and Michael Franti, thank you for writing great music that helped me write a good book.

To the birds outside my window, you make me very happy. I'll feed you millet and seeds always.

And finally, to my fans, and to everyone who has ever wanted to change their life but didn't know how, everything I do I do for you.

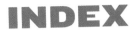

INDEX

family, 17
farmers' markets, 158
fasting, 112–16, 198
fats, 154–55
fermented foods, 153
Field Roast Grain Meat
    Company, 152
Fitzgerald, Randall, 131
flour, 151
Food and Drug Administration
    (FDA), 15
food combining, 99
food dehydrator, 156–57
food labeling, 147–49
food processor, 156
foodborne illness, 80
forgiveness, 199
free radicals, 32
Freedman, Rory, viii–ix
Freston, Kathy, 85, 161
frozen foods, 159
fruit, 36, 150–51
Fuhrman, Joe, 68

G
gadgets, 157
Gannon, Sharon, 127–29
Gardein, 152
gardening, 158–59
genetics, 10–11
Gershon, Michael, 92
GI Handbook (Ravage), 46
ginger baths, 139
global warming, 16, 81
glucose, 44–45
gluten-free foods, 52–55, 150
glycemic index, 46–47
greenhouse gases, 81

H
Harvard University, 125
heart disease, 9, 64–65
Hendel, Barbara, 30
Hertel, Hans Ulrich, 156
high-fructose corn syrup
    (HFCS), 148
Hippocrates Health Institute, 30,
    48, 113, 173
hormones, 76
hot dogs, 79

Hundred-Year Lie, The
    (Fitzgerald), 131
Hyman, Mark, 54–55

I
In Defense of Food (Pollan), 13
inflammation, 50–52
ingredient lists, 147–49
insulin resistance, 44–45
intestines, 91–92
iron, 70
irritable bowel syndrome
    (IBS), 103

J
juice, 105–8, 110, 112
    recipes, 207
juicers, 108–9
Junger, Alejandro, 77–78, 96–98

K
kapalabhati breathing, 137
ketosis, 78
knives, 156

L
Life, David, 129
Life's DHA Omega 3, 172
Lightlife, 152
Link, Lilli B., 50–52, 73–75
Lipman, Frank, 169–71
litmus paper, 24
liver, 43, 94–97
Living Foods for Optimum Health
    (Clement), 113
lutein, 33
lycopene, 33
lymph, 130
lymphatic drainage massage, 138

M
macrobiotics, 38
main course recipes, 217–21
Malkan, Stacy, 132–34
massage, 138–39
masticating juicers, 108–9
McGovern Report, 15
meat, 79–81
Meatless Monday campaign,
    71, 85

meat substitutes, 86, 152
meditation, 125–26
mercury, 102
microwaves, 156
milk, 71–73
minerals, 25–26
Mitchell, Joni, 11
money, 16, 157
monosodium glutamate
    (MSG), 148
MSM, 167
mucus, 92–93
Mucusless Diet Healing Program
    (Ehret), 93
multivitamins, 172

N
naps, 141
National Dairy Council, 71
neti pot, 136–37
New Glucose Revolution (Brand-
    Miller and Foster-Powell), 46
nut milk bag, 156
nutritional yeast, 153
nuts, 152, 156

O
oil, 155
omega-3 fatty acids, 51, 172
Oprah, 203
Ornish, Dean, vi–vii, 64
osteoporosis, 26
oxygen, 28–30

P
Pacelle, Wayne, 82–84
Pachauri, Rajendra, 81
parabens, 133
Pew Commission on Industrial
    Farm Animal Production, 83
pH, 21–26
phthalates, 132–33
phytonutrients, 33, 167
Pick, Marcelle, 101
Pollan, Michael, 13, 16
poop, 90–91, 102
Pottenger, Francis, 28
pregnancy, 56
preservatives, 149

Prevention of Farm Animal Cruelty
      Act, 84
Preventive Medicine Research
      Institute, ix
probiotics, 91–92, 166–67
processed meats, 79
protein, 68–70, 74
protein, plants high in, 70
protein powders, 167

Q
quercetin, 33

R
radiation, 121
raw food, 28–29
raw snacks, 154
rebounder, 130, 199
recipes
    desserts, 222
    juices and smoothies, 207
    main courses, 217–21
    salads and dressings, 208–13
    sauces, 216
    soups, 214–16
recombinant bovine growth
      hormone (rBGH), 76
reflex sympathetic dystrophy, 87
Reiki, 138–39
resources, 224–26
resveratrol, 33
rheumatoid arthritis, 18
Roth, Gabrielle, 126

S
Sacks, Stefanie, 147–49
sadhana, 127–28
salad recipes, 208–13
sauce recipes, 216
saunas, 139
seasonings, 153
seaweed, 153
seeds, 152
self-care, 123–24
Servan-Schreiber, David, 45
shopping list, 149–50
sinus problems, 136
Skin Deep database, 133–34
sleep, 140–41
slicing tools, 156

smoothie recipes, 207
smoothies, 111–12
snacks, 154
sodium, 74
soup, 150
soup recipes, 214–16
Southall, Ginger, 48
soy, 86
spirulina, 167
sprouts, 195
squatting, 98
steam baths, 139
stevia, 151
stress, 23
strokes, 9
sugar, 41–51
sunscreen, 170
Sunshine Veggie Burgers, 152
superfoods, 167
SUPERLOVE, 112
supplements, 165
sweat, 130
sweeteners, 148, 151

T
techno detox, 191
therapeutic baths, 139–40
time, 16–17
tongue scraping, 197
Toss It, 146
toxins, 131
trans fats, 51, 155
traveling, 200–201
triclosan, 132
20 Questions, 179
21-Day Cleanse, 177–205
    day 1 to 21, 184–205
    sample week, 181–82
    20 Questions, 179
    wean week, 180
twin gear juicers, 108–9

U
UltraMind Solution (Hyman), 55
United Nations, 81
US Department of Agriculture, 10,
      15, 42

V
vacuum sealer, 157

Vasey, Christopher, 34
veganism. See vegetarianism
Veganomicon (Moskowitz), 152
vegetables, 149–50
Vegetarian Passport, 201
vegetarianism
    benefits of, 10–11, 61–63
    protein and, 67–69
    eating out, 161
    traveling, 200–201
vision boards, 202–3
vitamin B12, 69, 168
vitamin C, 74
vitamin D, 168–71
vitamins, 32, 172
Vita-Mix, 111

W
Warburg, Otto, 28
water filters, 119–20
water, 29–30, 117–20
wean week, 180
weight-bearing exercise, 74
Weil, Andrew, 137
wheatgrass, 110
Wheatgrass Book, The
      (Wigmore), 110
wheatgrass implants, 94–95
Williamson, Marianne, 125
Women's Healthy Eating and
      Living study, 65
Women's Intervention Nutrition
      Study, 65
World Health Organization, 9

Y
yacón syrup, 151
yeast, 101–2
yoga, 129
yogurt, 91–92
Young Living Essential Oils, 135

Z
zeaxanthin, 33